# Human
# Reproductive
# Biology

Sylvia S. Mader

# Human Reproductive Biology

**wcb**
**Wm. C. Brown Co. Publishers**
*Dubuque, Iowa*

**wcb group**

**Wm. C. Brown**
*Chairman of the Board*
**Mark C. Falb**
*Executive Vice-President*

**wcb**

**Wm. C. Brown Company Publishers, College Division**

**Lawrence E. Cremer**
*President*
**David Wm. Smith**
*Vice-President, Marketing*
**E. F. Jogerst**
*Vice-President, Cost Analyst*
**David A. Corona**
*Assistant Vice-President, Production Development and Design*
**James L. Romig**
*Executive Editor*
**Marcia H. Stout**
*Marketing Manager*
**William A. Moss**
*Production Editorial Manager*
**Marilyn A. Phelps**
*Manager of Design*
**Mary M. Heller**
*Visual Research Manager*

Printed in the United States of America
10   9   8   7   6   5

*To my sister, Rhetta,
for her constant support*

# Contents

Preface   ix

1   **Inheritance**   **1**

1   Chromosomes and Chromosomal Inheritance   3
2   Genes and Autosomal Genetic Inheritance   24
3   Sex-Linked Inheritance   46
4   Biochemical Genetics   56
5   Modern Genetic Concerns   70

2   **Human Reproduction**   **83**

6   Secondary Sex Characteristics   85
7   Male Reproductive Anatomy   101
8   Female Reproductive Anatomy   113
9   Human Sexuality   127
10   Orgasm and Fertilization   142
11   Development and Birth   156
12   Birth Control and Infertility   174
13   Venereal Disease   191

3   **Evolution, Behavior, and Population**   **209**

14   Evolution of Sexual Reproduction   211
15   Biology of Sexual Behavior   224
16   Human Population   236

Epilogue   253
Appendix   255
Glossary   259
Index   271

# Preface

This book presents human reproduction from the biological point of view. As such, it suggests in Part 1 that the purpose of reproduction is the passage of DNA, the genetic material, from one generation to another. DNA makes up the genes that lie within the chromosomes and chromosomal inheritance is discussed prior to genetic inheritance. Sexual reproduction assures that the genotype of the offspring will differ from the genotype of either parent. The chances of an offspring receiving a certain combination of genes may be calculated and this is particularly helpful when the offspring might receive a gene that causes a genetic disease. Both theoretical scientists and medical practitioners are presently emphasizing that many human illnesses are actually genetic diseases that can possibly be prevented. Techniques are available today and perhaps soon more will be available to control and to cure genetic diseases. The hope for cures lies in modern genetic research including genetic engineering, both of which are outlined in this book.

In Part 2, hormone action is explained before male and female reproductive anatomy and physiology are presented in depth. Then, psychological aspects of human sexuality are presented before sexual response is explained biologically. Following a description of fertilization, the major biological events of embryonic and fetal development are outlined. A discussion of birth control procedures and devices emphasizes the effectiveness and the side effects of each method. Signs, symptoms, and cures of venereal diseases are reviewed because they are the most prevalent of all contagious diseases today. It is hoped that a biological understanding of human reproduction will give young people a means of control over their lives that they may not have had before.

In Part 3, the evolution of sexual reproduction is presumed to have increased biological fitness. That is, it is assumed that sexual reproduction has increased the likelihood of survival and propagation. Biologically fit organisms are adapted to their environment and this adaptation includes anatomical, physiological, and behavioral adaptation. Sociobiology suggests that human reproductive behavior evolved to ensure the passage of genes. This tenet is examined. Even if human reproductive behavior is ultimately controlled by genes, it is immediately controlled by the nervous system. Accumulating data suggest a dimorphic development of the brain that might affect human behavior even though much of human behavior is learned.

The reproductive drive in humans has resulted in a very large human population. The fact that population growth might possibly be leveling off in the developed countries suggests a growing awareness of the concept of carrying capacity. Population growth in the underdeveloped countries continues to increase and the problems of population growth are examined.

This text is most appropriate for use by nonscience students who would like a biological understanding of human reproduction. The three parts of the book may be studied in whatever sequence the instructor desires. It is hoped that the student will be assisted in the learning process by various aids. Important terms which appear in boldface are also listed at the end of each chapter and are defined in the glossary. Charts summarize and highlight important points. Illustrations are carefully correlated with the text, and diagrams are used to clarify the more detailed concepts. Each chapter ends with a set of study questions, and each part has a list of further readings.

The author wishes to acknowledge the help of Dr. Clifford J. Dennis, Biology department, University of Wisconsin-Whitewater; Dr. Nancy Harvilla-Ellis, department of Physiology and Health Sciences, Ball State University; Dr. Richard Armstrong, Biology department, Santa Barbara City College; Dr. Robert Beamon, chairperson, Biology department, Hillsborough Community College; Dr. David Robertshaw, department of Physiology, Indiana University at Bloomington; and Ms. Marian Z. Grabowski, R.N., department of Biology, University of Miami at Coral Gabels who reviewed the manuscript and provided many helpful suggestions. The illustrations were all originally drawn and skillfully rendered by Lydia Greselin. My typist, Adelle Robinson, was both competent and faithful. Finally, many thanks to the personnel of Wm. C. Brown Company, who carefully and cheerfully guided all aspects of production.

# *Part* **1 Inheritance**

# Chromosomes and Chromosomal Inheritance

Every human being is made up of millions of cells. Figure 1.1 shows a generalized cell which can be divided for convenience into two parts: the cytoplasm and the nucleus. The **cytoplasm**, sometimes defined as the liquid portion of the cell, surrounds the central **nucleus** and contains various small bodies called organ-

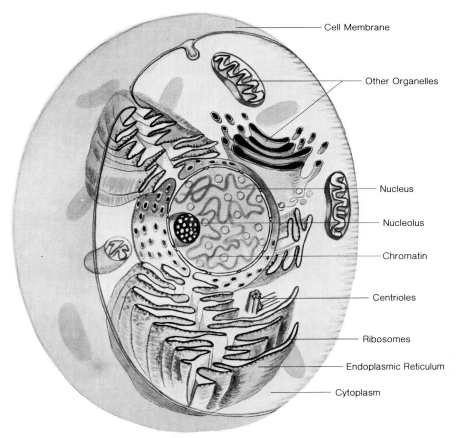

Figure 1.1   A cell, the smallest unit of life, in a multicellular organism contains many different organelles. (After Mader, *Inquiry into Life,* 2d edition.)

elles. Each organelle has a specific support function for the cell and those of interest to us will be discussed in Chapter 4. Inside the nucleus are the **chromosomes**, filamentous structures, each of which carries a variety of genes. **Genes** determine what the cell is like and what the individual is like. In a non-dividing cell the chromosomes are indistinct and diffuse, but in a dividing cell the chromosomes become short and thick and may be counted. Normal humans contain 23 pairs of chromosomes, or 46 chromosomes altogether, in each nucleus.

*Karyotype.* A cell may be photographed just prior to division so that a picture of the chromosomes is obtained. The chromosomes may be cut out of the picture and arranged by pairs (fig. 1.2).

Pairs of chromosomes are recognized by the fact that they are of the same size and have the same general appearance. Chromosomes may also be stained to show that pairs have similar banding patterns (fig. 1.3).

The resulting display of pairs of chromosomes is called a **karyotype** (fig. 1.4). Although both male and female have 23 pairs of chromosomes, one of

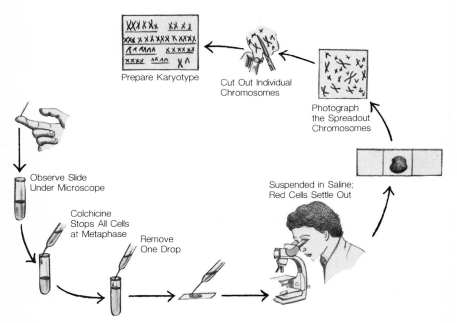

Prepare Karyotype

Cut Out Individual Chromosomes

Photograph the Spreadout Chromosomes

Observe Slide Under Microscope

Suspended in Saline; Red Cells Settle Out

Colchicine Stops All Cells at Metaphase

Remove One Drop

Figure 1.2 A karyotype is an arrangement of chromosome photos, by pairs.

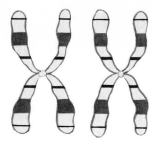

Figure 1.3  Banding shows that pairs of chromosomes are similarly constructed.

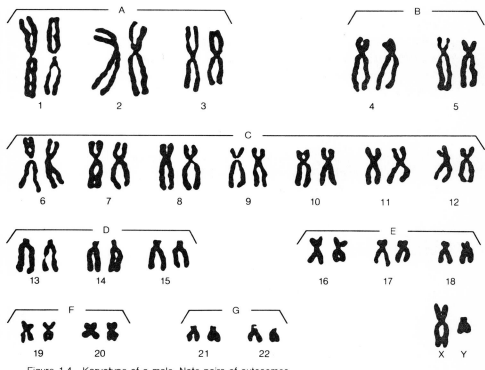

Figure 1.4  Karyotype of a male. Note pairs of autosomes that are numbered from 1–22 and one pair of sex chromosomes, X and Y.

these pairs is of unequal length in the male. The larger chromosome of this pair is called the X and the smaller is called the Y. Females have two X chromosomes in their karyotype. The X and Y chromosomes are called the **sex chromosomes** because they contain the genes that determine sex. The other chromosomes, known as **autosomes,** include all the pairs of chromosomes except the X and Y chromosomes. Notice that each pair of autosomes in the human karyotype is numbered.

## Life Cycle

The human life cycle requires **sexual reproduction** in which the **sperm** of the male fertilizes the **egg** in the female; the resulting **zygote** develops into the newborn infant which grows to be an adult (fig. 1.5). Two types of cell division occur during the human life cycle. **Meiosis** occurs as a part of **gametogenesis,** the production of **gametes**, which is a term used collectively to mean the sperm and egg. Because of meiosis, the sperm contains 23 chromosomes and the egg contains 23 chromosomes. The zygote contains 23 pairs of chromosomes; one of each pair was contributed by the father and one of each pair was contributed by the mother.

The second type of cell division, called **mitosis**, occurs whenever growth takes place, such as when the zygote develops into a newborn. The zygote has 46 chromosomes and as a result of mitosis every cell in the body has 46 chromosomes. Each cell in the body has a copy of the chromosomes and genes originally contributed by the parents. Offspring tend to resemble their parents. This may be explained by the fact that the parents and child share common chromosomes and genes.

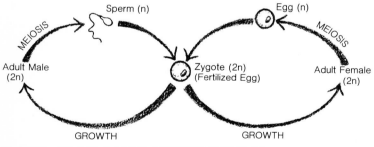

Figure 1.5   Life cycle of humans requires two types of cell division: meiosis and mitosis. (After Mader, *Inquiry into Life,* 2d edition.)

# Cell Division

Mitosis

*Mitosis* is cell division in which the chromosome number stays constant. The original cell, called the **mother** cell, has 46 chromosomes in humans and the two **daughter**, or resulting, cells also have 46 chromosomes. When a cell has the full number of possible chromosomes, it is said to have the **diploid**, or *2N* **number** of chromosomes. Mitosis, then, is cell division in which 2N———> 2N.

Figure 1.6 shows a diagram of a mother cell that for simplicity's sake has only two pairs of chromosomes. Notice that each chromosome is duplicated and that each has two identical portions called chromatids. During mitosis, the chromatids separate and one chromatid from each duplicated chromosome goes to each daughter cell. Thus, each daughter cell will have the same number and kinds of chromosomes as the mother cell. Before the daughter cells can divide again, the chromosomes must duplicate to have two chromatids.

Figure 1.7 diagrams the process of mitosis as it occurs in somatic cells. The process actually requires several stages during which the nuclear membrane disappears and a spindle apparatus with spindle fibers forms (fig. 1.8). The chromosomes are attached to the spindle fibers by structures called centromeres and the chromosomes move to the center of the mother cell before the centromere splits and the chromatids separate. The separated chromatids, now called daughter chromosomes, move away from each other into the newly forming daughter cells.

Mitosis is the type of cell division required for growth and repair of body cells. The process of mitosis assures that each cell in the body has the same number and kinds of chromosomes and genes.

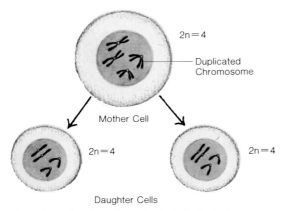

Figure 1.6   Overview of mitosis. During mitosis, the chromatids of a duplicated chromosome separate so that the daughter cells have the same number and kinds of chromosomes as the mother cell.

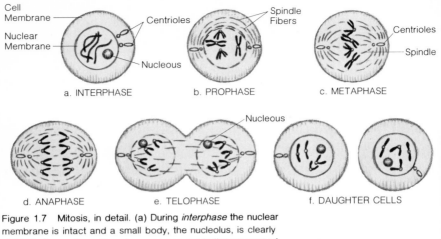

a. INTERPHASE  b. PROPHASE  c. METAPHASE

d. ANAPHASE  e. TELOPHASE  f. DAUGHTER CELLS

Figure 1.7   Mitosis, in detail. (a) During *interphase* the nuclear membrane is intact and a small body, the nucleolus, is clearly visible in the nucleus. The chromosomes are in the process of duplicating as are the centrioles, organelles associated with the formation of the spindle apparatus. (b) During *prophase* the nuclear membrane and nucleolus are disappearing and the spindle fibers are appearing as the centrioles move apart. The chromosomes are distinct and duplicated. (c) During *metaphase* the chromosomes are lined up at the middle of the spindle apparatus. (d) During *anaphase* the chromatids separate and the resulting daughter chromosomes move apart. (e) During *telophase* the nuclear membrane and nucleolus are reappearing and the spindle fibers are disappearing. Furrowing of the cell membrane divides the cytoplasm between (f) two daughter cells. (After Mader, *Inquiry into Life,* 2d edition.)

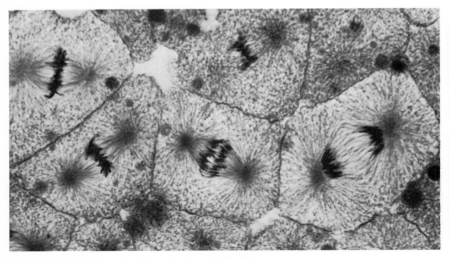

Figure 1.8   Photograph of cells undergoing mitosis. (Source: Courtesy of the Macmillan Science Co., Inc., Chicago, IL 60620.)

## Meiosis

*Meiosis* is cell division in which the chromosome number is halved. In humans, the mother cell has 46 chromosomes, but at the completion of meiosis the daughter cells have 23 chromosomes. Half the chromosome number is called the **haploid**, or *N*, **number** of chromosomes. Meiosis is cell division in which $2N \longrightarrow N$.

Meiosis (fig. 1.9) requires two cell divisions for completion; consequently, there are four daughter cells, each having the haploid number of chromosomes. Before meiosis, similar duplicated chromosomes in the mother cell come together in pairs. During the first meiotic division, the pairs of duplicated chromosomes separate, resulting in daughter cells with only one of each chromosomal pair. During the second division, chromatids separate; thus, the four daughter cells have half the number of chromosomes as the mother cell and one of each kind of chromosome as compared to the original mother cell.

Figures 1.10 and 1.11 show the process of meiosis in detail. The process actually requires several stages. Each series of stages occurs twice: once during meiosis I (fig. 1.10) and again during meiosis II (fig. 1.11). Whereas mitosis is the cell division for growth and repair, meiosis occurs only during the production

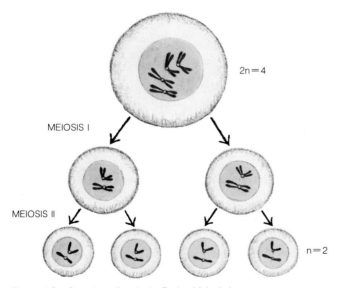

MEIOSIS I

MEIOSIS II

$2n = 4$

$n = 2$

Figure 1.9  Overview of meiosis. During Meiosis I, chromosome pairs separate so that the daughter cells have one of each kind of duplicated chromosome. During Meiosis II, chromatids separate so that the four resulting daughter cells have one-half the number and one of each kind of chromosome as the original mother cell. (After Mader, *Inquiry into Life,* 2d edition.)

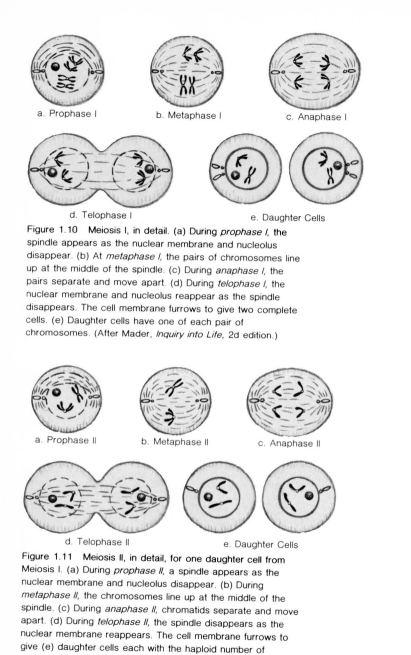

a. Prophase I

b. Metaphase I

c. Anaphase I

d. Telophase I

e. Daughter Cells

Figure 1.10    Meiosis I, in detail. (a) During *prophase I*, the spindle appears as the nuclear membrane and nucleolus disappear. (b) At *metaphase I*, the pairs of chromosomes line up at the middle of the spindle. (c) During *anaphase I*, the pairs separate and move apart. (d) During *telophase I*, the nuclear membrane and nucleolus reappear as the spindle disappears. The cell membrane furrows to give two complete cells. (e) Daughter cells have one of each pair of chromosomes. (After Mader, *Inquiry into Life*, 2d edition.)

a. Prophase II

b. Metaphase II

c. Anaphase II

d. Telophase II

e. Daughter Cells

Figure 1.11    Meiosis II, in detail, for one daughter cell from Meiosis I. (a) During *prophase II*, a spindle appears as the nuclear membrane and nucleolus disappear. (b) During *metaphase II*, the chromosomes line up at the middle of the spindle. (c) During *anaphase II*, chromatids separate and move apart. (d) During *telophase II*, the spindle disappears as the nuclear membrane reappears. The cell membrane furrows to give (e) daughter cells each with the haploid number of chromosomes. (After Mader, *Inquiry into Life*, 2d edition.)

of gametes. The production of sperm cells in males is called **spermatogenesis**; production of the egg cell in females is called **oogenesis.**

*Spermatogenesis.* Figure 1.12 shows meiosis as it occurs in the testes (p. 102) of males during *spermatogenesis*, or sperm production (fig. 1.14a). Figure 1.12 is diagrammatic and for simplicity's sake the mother cell has only one pair of autosomes and the sex chromosomes, *X* and *Y.* The first set of daughter cells has only one autosome and one sex chromosome because the pairs of chromosomes have separated. Separation of chromatids in the next division results

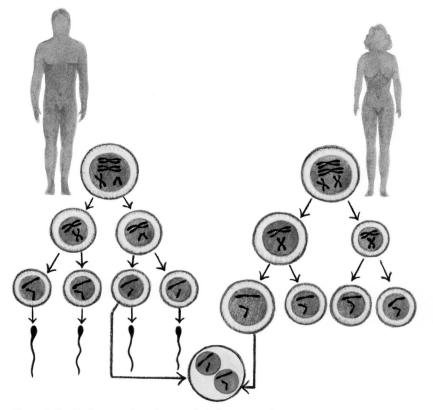

Figure 1.12 Each spermatogonium results in four sperm. In this diagram, the mother cell is shown as having one autosomal pair (normally there are twenty-two pairs) and the sex chromosomes X and Y. Note that following meiosis, two sperm carry an X chromosome and two sperm carry a Y chromosome.

Figure 1.13 Each oogenesis results in one egg. In this diagram, the mother cell is shown as having one autosomal pair (normally there are 22 pairs) and 2 X sex chromosomes. Note that following meiosis, the egg carries an X chromosome.

in four daughter cells, each of which has the haploid number of chromosomes. Notice that two sperm carry an *X* chromosome and two sperm carry a *Y* chromosome.

*Oogenesis.* Figure 1.13 diagrammatically shows meiosis in females where meiosis is a part of *oogenesis*. Oogenesis, which occurs in the ovaries (p. 114), differs from spermatogenesis in that the first meiotic division results in one viable daughter cell and one **polar body**. A polar body is a much smaller cell that

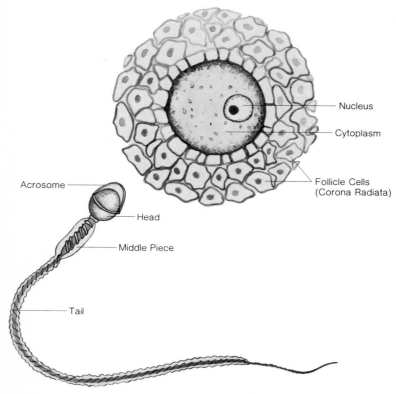

Figure 1.14    The egg is spherical and much larger than the sperm due to the fact that it contains a great deal of cytoplasm. The outer membrane of the egg is convoluted and often surrounded by adhering cells collectively called the corona radiata. The mature sperm, which measures 1/500 inch, consists of a head region, middle piece, and tail region. The flattened and almond-shaped head contains the nucleus, very little cytoplasm, and a caplike acrosome at the anterior end. The acrosome contains enzymes that are capable of digesting away the outer covering of the egg. The middle piece produces the energy that allows the tail to move back and forth, accounting for the ability of the sperm to swim.

is believed to be nonfunctional. The second meiotic division also results in one daughter cell and one polar body. Only the daughter cell containing most of the cytoplasm matures into an egg (fig. 1.14b) and thus females produce only one egg per oogenesis. Note that because the mother cell had the sex chromosomes XX, the egg must carry an X chromosome.

Egg production occurs once a month in females, while sperm production occurs continuously in males. At the time of ejaculation during intercourse, males emit as many as 400 million or more sperm (p. 103).

## Chromosomal Inheritance

As mentioned previously , the individual normally receives 22 autosomal chromosomes and one sex chromosome from each parent. The sex of the newborn child is determined by whether a Y- or X- bearing sperm fertilizes the egg. While it is obvious that there is a 50 percent chance, all other factors being equal, of having a girl and a 50 percent chance of having a boy, it is possible to illustrate this probability by doing a **Punnett Square** (fig. 1.15). In the square, all possible sperm are lined up on one side; all possible eggs are lined up on the other side (or vice versa), and every possible mating is considered. When this is done with regard to sex chromosomes, the results show one female to each male. Thus, the chance of bearing a male offspring is just as great as that of bearing a female.

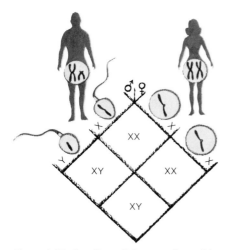

Figure 1.15   In a Punnett Square, all possible sperm fertilize all possible eggs so that the chances of having a particular offspring can be determined. Here sperm and eggs are shown as carrying only a sex chromosome; actually, of course, they also carry 22 autosomes. The offspring (located within the squares) are either male or female depending on whether they received an X or Y from the male parent.

Sometimes individuals are born with either too many or too few chromosomes. It is possible also that even though there is the correct number of chromosomes, one chromosome may be defective in some way. Both autosomal and sex chromosome abnormalities do occur.

Autosomal Chromosomal Abnormalities

The most common autosomal abnormality is seen in individuals who have **Down's Syndrome** (fig. 1.16). A **syndrome** is a group of physical signs or symptoms that always occur together and characterize a medical condition. Down's syndrome is sometimes called mongolism because the eyes of the

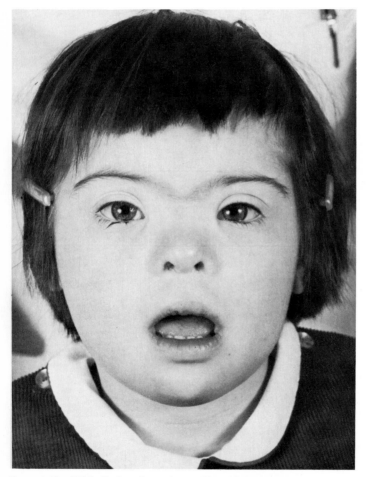

Figure 1.16  Child with Down's syndrome. (From M. Bartalos and T.A. Baramski, *Medical Cytogenetics*, 1967, The Williams & Wilkins, Co.)

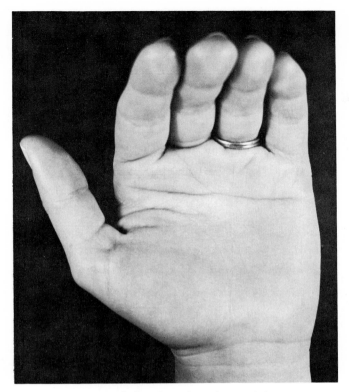

Figure 1.17  Persons with Down's syndrome have a simian
crease. (Source: A.M. Winchester.)

person seem to have an oriental-like fold, but this term is not considered scientific.
Other characteristics are short stature; stubby fingers; a wide gap between the
first and second toes; a large, fissured tongue; a round head; a palm crease,
the so-called simian line (fig. 1.17), and, unfortunately, mental retardation that
can sometimes be severe.

*Nondisjunction.*   Persons with Down's syndrome usually have three number 21
chromosomes because the egg had two number 21 chromosomes instead of
one. Either the chromosome pair (fig. 1.18a) or the chromatids (fig. 1.18b) failed
to separate completely and instead went into the same daughter cell. Either of
these occurrences is called **nondisjunction**. It would appear that nondisjunction
is most apt to occur in the older female since children with Down's syndrome
are usually born to women over age forty. If the older woman wishes to know
whether or not her unborn child is affected by Down's syndrome, she may elect
to undergo **amniocentesis** (fig. 1.19). In this procedure a small amount of
*amniotic fluid* surrounding the developing fetus in the uterus is withdrawn, and

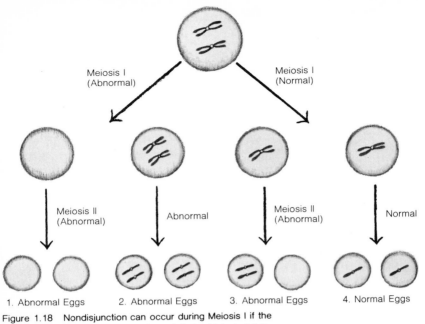

Figure 1.18   Nondisjunction can occur during Meiosis I if the
chromosome pairs fail to separate and during Meiosis II if the
chromatids fail to separate completely. In either case, the
abnormal eggs carry an extra chromosome.

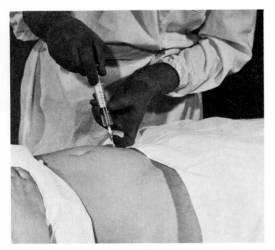

Figure 1.19   During amniocentesis, a large needle is inserted
through the abdominal wall into the uterus.

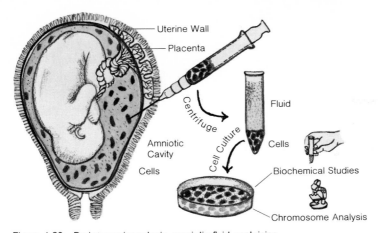

Figure 1.20   During amniocentesis, amniotic fluid containing
fetal cells is withdrawn. Chromosome analysis and biochemical
studies can determine if the offspring has certain types of
defects. (After Friedmann, Theodore, "Prenatal Diagnosis of
Genetic Disease," *Scientific American*, Nov. 1971.)

the fetal cells within the fluid are examined for genetic defects (fig. 1.20). A
karyotype of the chromosomes indicates whether or not the unborn child has
Down's syndrome. If so, the couple may elect to continue or to abort the pregnancy.

*Deletion.*    Another chromosomal abnormality called deletion is responsible for
a syndrome known as **Cri du Chat.** The condition derives its name from French,
and affected individuals meow like a kitten when they cry. More important, perhaps, is the fact that they tend to have a small head with malformations of the
face and body (fig. 1.21) . Mental defectiveness usually causes retarded development. Chromosomal analysis shows that a portion of chromosome number
5 is missing (deleted), while the other number 5 chromosome is normal.

Sex Chromosome Abnormalities

Individuals are sometimes born with the sex chromosomes XO (Turner's syndrome), XXX (superfemale), XXY (Klinefelter's syndrome), and XYY (chart 1.1).
Individuals with a Y are always male no matter how many X chromosomes there
may be; however, at least one X chromosome is needed for survival. A fetus
with only a Y chromosome dies spontaneously before delivery.

Abnormal sex chromosome constituencies may result from nondisjunction
of the sex chromosomes during oogenesis or spermatogenesis. Nondisjunction
during oogenesis can lead to an egg with either two X chromosomes or no X
chromosomes.

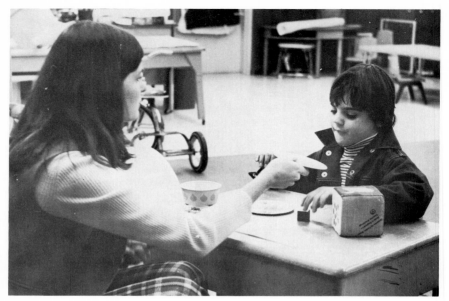

Figure 1.21   Child with Cri du Chat syndrome receiving educational therapy. (Source: A.M. Winchester.)

**Chart 1.1**
Sex Chromosome Abnormalities

| Name | Chromosomes | Frequency/Live Births |
|------|-------------|----------------------|
| Turner's | XO | 1/3,500 |
| Superfemale | XXX | 1/1,000 |
| Klinefelter's | XXY | 1/800 |
| --- | XYY | 1/700 |

When these eggs are fertilized with a normal sperm a superfemale, a male with Klinefelter's syndrome, or a female with Turner's syndrome can result. Non-disjunction during spermatogenesis can lead to a sperm that has no sex chromosome, both an X and a Y chromosome, two X chromosomes, or two Y chromosomes because nondisjunction can be caused by a failure of chromosomes to separate or by a failure of chromatids to separate completely (fig. 1.22). Fertilization of normal eggs with affected sperm can give a Turner female, Klinefelter male, a superfemale, or an XYY male.

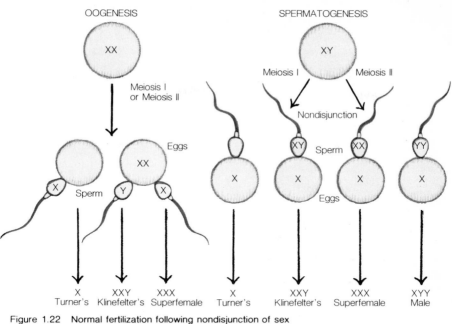

Figure 1.22   Normal fertilization following nondisjunction of sex chromosomes during the production of eggs and sperm could result in the syndromes noted.

## Abnormal Females

*Turner's syndrome.*   The XO individual has only one sex chromosome—an X; the O signifies the absence of the second sex chromosome. The ovaries never become functional and instead regress to ridges of white streaks. Because of this, females with Turner's syndrome do not undergo puberty; they do not menstruate; and there is a lack of breast development (fig. 1.23). Generally, these individuals have a stocky build, a webbed neck, and subnormal intelligence.

*Superfemale.*   It might be supposed that the XXX female with 47 chromosomes would be especially feminate, but this is not the case. Although there is a tendency toward mental retardation, most superfemales have no apparent physical abnormalities and many are fertile. Their children have a normal chromosome count; it has been suggested that the extra X chromosome is discarded during oogenesis.

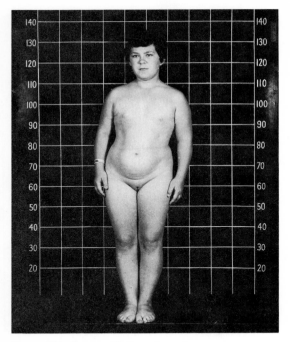

Figure 1.23   Person with Turner's syndrome.

## Abnormal Males

*Klinefelter's syndrome.*   Males with XXY sex chromosomes are male in general appearance, but their testes are underdeveloped and their breasts are often enlarged (fig. 1.24). Most of these individuals are sterile because the testes do not mature normally. Limbs of these men tend to be longer than average, their body hair is sparse, and many are mentally defective.

As a general rule, the greater the excess of X chromosomes, the greater the degree of mental abnormality. Individuals with the chromosomes XXXY, XXXXY, and so forth are severely retarded.

*XYY males.*   Afflicted males are usually taller than average (more than six feet tall), suffer from persistent acne, and tend to have barely normal intelligence. It is not known whether the subnormal intelligence is due to their chromosome makeup or whether their impulsive behavioral characteristics hinder their ability to learn. At one time, it was suggested that these men were likely to be criminally aggressive, but it has been shown that the incidence of this behavior is quite low.

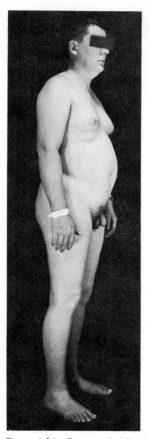

Figure 1.24   Person with Klinefelter's syndrome. (Source:
Courtesy of F.A. Davis Company, Philadelphia, and Dr. R.H.
Kampmeier.

---

## Summary

Human beings are made up of cells, each containing a nucleus with 46
chromosomes. A karyotype is a pictorial display showing the chromosomes
arranged in 22 pairs of autosomal chromosomes and 1 pair of sex
chromosomes. An individual with the sex chromosomes XX is a female and
one with the sex chromosomes XY is a male.

The human life cycle depends on sexual reproduction and two types of
cell divisions—mitosis, in which the chromosome number stays constant
(2N $\rightarrow$ 2N) and meiosis, in which the chromosome number is halved
(2N$\rightarrow$N). Mitosis occurs during growth and repair of cells and results in two
daughter cells each with 46 daughter chromosomes. Meiosis occurs during

gametogenesis, the production of sex cells, and results in four daughter cells each with 23 chromosomes, one of each pair. In males, meiosis is a part of spermatogenesis and in females it is a part of oogenesis. When the sperm fertilizes the egg during sexual reproduction, the resulting zygote has 46 chromosomes or 23 pairs. One of each chromosomal pair was derived from the sperm and one was derived from the egg.

Autosomal chromosome abnormalities commonly occur in humans due to nondisjunction and deletion; Down's and Cri du Chat syndrome are two examples. Sex chromosome abnormalities, such as Turner's syndrome and Klinefelter's syndrome, that are discussed in this chapter appear in Chart 1.1.

## Terms

amniocentesis
cell
  cytoplasm
  nucleus
  organelle
chromosomes
  autosomes
  centromere
  chromatid
  diploid (2N) number
  genes
  haploid (N) number
  sex chromosomes
Cri du Chat
Down's syndrome

gametes
  gametogenesis
karyotype
Klinefelter's syndrome
meiosis
  oogenesis
  polar body
  spermatogenesis
mitosis
nondisjunction
Punnett Square
superfemale
Turner's syndrome
XYY male
zygote

## Review

1. Redraw the life cycle of humans, including the processes of meiosis, mitosis, spermatogenesis, and oogenesis. Use the appropriate number to denote the chromosomal makeup of the structures.
2. Draw a generalized diagram for mitosis.
   (a) In each cell, put the notation 2N or N as appropriate.
   (b) Sketch an autosomal pair of chromosomes in the mother cell and show what happens to the chromosomes during the process of cell division.

3. Draw a generalized diagram for meiosis.
   (a) In each cell, put the notation 2N or N as appropriate.
   (b) Place and autosomal pair of chromosomes in the mother cell and show what happens to the chromosomes during the process of meiosis.
   (c) Since genes are carried on the chromosomes, put a gene designated as A on one of the autosomal chromosomes and a gene designated as a on the other. In terms of these letters, what two types of gametes are possible?

4. List several differences between mitosis and meiosis considering:
   (a) the purpose, (b) the occurrence in the body, (c) the number of divisions, (d) the number of daughter cells, (e) the number changes of the chromosomes, and (f) the resulting number of chromosomes in the daughter cells.

5. Diagram spermatogenesis and oogenesis. Note several differences between the two processes.

6. Name two inherited syndromes caused by autosomal chromosome abnormalities. State the abnormality in each and describe the appearance of the affected individual.

7. What is amniocentesis? How is it performed? What are its merits? How can a karyotype suggest that a baby will be abnormal at birth?

8. Name two conditions of sex chromosome abnormalities in females. What are the sex chromosomes for each? Describe the appearance of the individual for each.

9. Name two conditions of sex chromosome abnormalities in males. What are the sex chromosomes for each? Describe the appearance of the individual for each.

10. What is nondisjunction? Diagram autosomal nondisjunction showing sex chromosome nondisjunction for both spermatogenesis and oogenesis.

# 2    Genes and Autosomal Genetic Inheritance

*Genes*, the units of heredity that control specific characteristics of an individual, are arranged in a linear fashion within each chromosome. It is customary to designate a gene by a letter in terms of the specific characteristic it controls; a **dominant gene** is assigned a capital letter, while a **recessive gene** is given the same lowercase letter. In humans, for example, free ear lobes are dominant over attached ear lobes, so a suitable key would be: E for free ear lobes and e for attached ear lobes.

The individual has two genes for a characteristic if these genes are carried on autosomal chromosomes. The genes have a particular location on a particular chromosome; therefore, just as one of each pair of chromosomes is inherited from each parent, so one of each pair of genes is inherited from each parent.

Figure 2.1 shows three possible fertilizations and the resulting genetic make-up of the zygote and thus, the individual. In the first instance, the chromosome of both the sperm and egg carries an E. Consequently, the zygote and subsequent individual have the genes EE, which may be called a **pure dominant**[1] genotype (chart 2.1). The word **genotype** refers to the genes of the individual. A person with genotype EE obviously has free ear lobes. The physical appearance of the individual, in this case free ear lobes, is called the **phenotype.**

In the second fertilization, the zygote received two recessive genes (ee), and the genotype is called **pure recessive.**[2] An individual with this genotype has attached ear lobes. In the third fertilization, the resulting individual has the genes Ee, which is called a **hybrid**[3] genotype. A hybrid shows the dominant characteristic; thus, the phenotype of this individual is free ear lobes.

The examples above show that a dominant gene can cause a particular phenotype when contributed from only one parent. A recessive gene needs to be given from both parents to affect the phenotype.

Determining the Genotype of the Child

Many times parents would like to know what the chances are that an *individual* child will have a certain genotype and thus, a certain characteristic. If one of

1. Often called homozygous dominant.
2. Often called homozygous recessive.
3. Often called heterozygous.

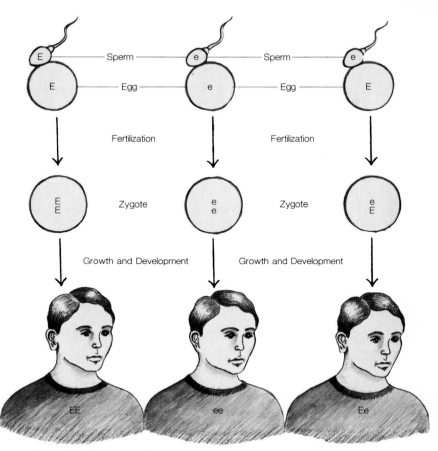

Figure 2.1 (a) If both sperm and egg carry a dominant gene designated as an E, then the individual has the gene type EE and the phenotype free earlobes. (b) If both sperm and egg carry a recessive gene designated by e, then the individual has the genotype ee and the phenotype attached earlobes. (c) If the sperm carries a recessive gene, e, and the egg carries a dominant gene, E, then the individual has the genotype Ee and the phenotype free earlobes.

## Chart 2.1

| Genotype (in letters) | Genotype (in words) | Phenotype |
|---|---|---|
| EE | Pure dominant | Unattached ear lobes |
| ee | Pure recessive | Attached ear lobes |
| Ee | Hybrid | Unattached ear lobes |

the parents is pure dominant (EE), it is obvious that the chances of a child with free ear lobes are 100 percent, because this parent has only a capital E to pass on to the offspring. On the other hand, if both parents are pure recessive (ee), there is a 100 percent chance that each child will have attached lobes. However, there are instances in which the expected phenotype is not so easily ascertained. Suppose both parents are hybrids, then what are the chances that a child will have free ear lobes or attached ear lobes? To solve a problem of this type, it is customary to first indicate the genotype of the parents and their possible gametes:

Genotypes:              Ee × Ee

Gametes:                E,e   E,e

*Second*, a Punnett Square (fig. 2.2) is used to determine the phenotype ratio among the offspring when all possible sperm are given an equal chance to fertilize all possible eggs. The sperm are lined up along one side of the square, while the eggs are lined up along the other side of the square (or vice versa). The ratio among the offspring in this case is 3:1 (three children with free ear lobes to one with attached ear lobes). This means that there is a ¾ chance

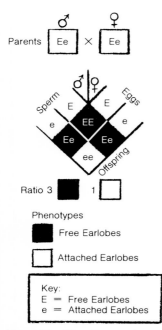

Figure 2.2   When the parents are hybrids, each child has a 75 percent chance of having the dominant phenotype and a 25 percent chance of having the recessive phenotype.

(75 percent) for each child to have free ear lobes and a ¼ chance (25 percent) for each child to have attached ear lobes.

Another mating of particular interest is that between a hybrid (Ee) and a pure recessive (ee). In this case, the Punnett Square operation (fig. 2.3) shows that the ratio among the offspring is 1:1 and the chance of the dominant or recessive phenotype is ½ or 50 percent.

Chart 2.2 summarizes the expected results from the matings mentioned above.

Normal Characteristics

Chart 2.3 lists several normal characteristics of human beings that are known to be either autosomal recessive or dominant, and figure 2.4 shows some of these pictorially. Each child has a 75 percent chance of having the dominant phenotype if the two parents are hybrids and a 50 percent chance if one parent is hybrid and the other is recessive. Each child has a 25 percent chance of having the recessive phenotype if the parents are hybrids and a 50 percent chance if one parent is a hybrid and the other is pure recessive.

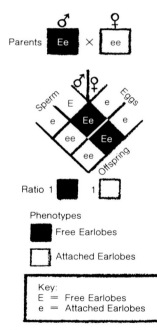

Figure 2.3  When one parent is hybrid and the other is recessive, each child has a 50 percent chance of having the dominant phenotype and a 50 percent chance of having the recessive phenotype.

## Chart 2.2
Possible Matings

| Genotype of Parents | Chance of Dominant Phenotype (percent) | Chance of Recessive Phenotype (percent) |
|---|---|---|
| EE × EE | 100 | 0 |
| EE × Ee | 100 | 0 |
| EE × ee | 100 | 0 |
| Ee × Ee | 75 | 25 |
| Ee × ee | 50 | 50 |
| ee × ee | 0 | 100 |

## Chart 2.3
Human Genetic Traits

| Trait | Dominant | Recessive |
|---|---|---|
| Earlobes | Free | Attached |
| Hair color | Dark | Light |
| Eye color | Dark | Light |
| Tongue | Roller | Nonroller |
| Freckles | Present | Absent |
| Widow's peak | Present | Absent |
| Hitchhiker's thumb | Present | Absent |
| Interlocking fingers | Right over left | Left over right |
| Nose shape | Convex | Straight |
| Dimples | Present | Absent |
| Bent little finger | Bent | Straight |
| Handedness | Right | Left |
| Second finger | Shorter than fourth | Longer than fourth |
| Mid-digital hair | Present | Absent |
| PTC* | Taster | Nontaster |

*A chemical phenylthiocarbamide is an antithyroid drug that prevents the thyroid from incorporating iodine into the thyroid hormone. The ability to taste PTC is associated with pathology of the thyroid gland.

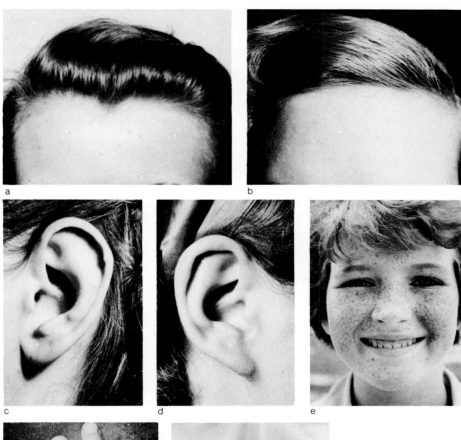

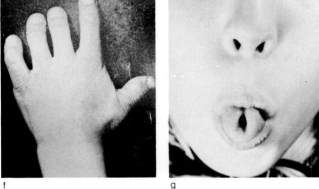

Figure 2.4 Common inherited characteristics in human beings.
Widow's peak (a) is dominant over continuous hairline (b).
Unattached earlobe (c) is dominant over attached earlobe (d).
Freckles (e) are dominant over no freckles. Short fingers
(f) are dominant over long fingers. Ability to roll the tongue
(g) is dominant over inability to roll the tongue. (Source: A.M.
Winchester.)

## Chart 2.4

Estimated Incidence and Prevalence of Selected Birth Defects, U.S.A., 1976

| Condition | Newly Affected | Under Age 20 with Condition |
|---|---|---|
| Anencephaly | 3,100 | |
| Spina bifida and/or hydrocephalus | 6,200 | 53,000 |
| Cleft lip and/or cleft palate | 4,300 | 71,000 |
| Congenital heart disease | 24,800 | 248,000 |
| Clubfoot | 9,300 | 149,000 |
| Congenital dislocation of hip | 3,100 | 50,000 |
| Polydactyly (extra fingers and toes) | 9,300 | 184,000 |
| Syndactyly | 1,000 | 21,000 |
| Cystic fibrosis | 2,000 | 10,000 |
| Hemophilia | 1,200 | 12,400 |
| Phenylketonuria | 310 | 3,100 |
| Sickle-cell anemia | 1,200 | 16,000 |
| Tay-Sachs disease | 30 | 100 |
| Thalassemia (Cooley's anemia) | 70 | 1,000 |
| Diabetes | .. | 90,000 |
| Down's syndrome | 5,100 | 44,000 |
| Other mental retardation of prenatal origin | 44,000 | 800,000 |

*Fatal soon after birth.
**Late-appearing birth defects.
Note: Some children have more than one kind of birth defect; hence the
total number with one or more of the specific defects cited is smaller
than the sum of the number for each condition.
(Source: HEW.)

## Genetic Diseases

It is now apparent that many illnesses of human beings are genetic in origin.
**Genetic diseases** are medical conditions that are caused by genes inherited
from the parents. Some of these conditions are controlled by autosomal dominant
or recessive genes. Several of these conditions and their frequencies are listed
in chart 2.4.

Recessive Genetic Diseases

Figure 2.5 shows a typical **pedigree chart** of a family tree for a recessive
genetic disease.[4] It is obvious that a genetic condition is recessive when an
afflicted child is born to parents who appear to be normal. Parents with a hybrid
genotype, those who carry a hidden faulty gene, are called **carriers**. When a

4. For other examples, see Appendix A.

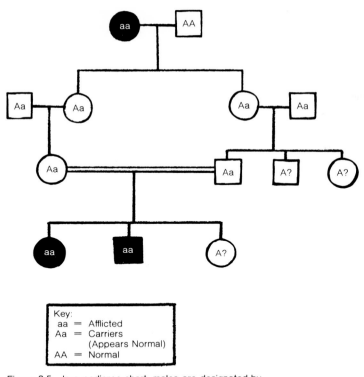

Key:
aa = Afflicted
Aa = Carriers
      (Appears Normal)
AA = Normal

Figure 2.5   In a pedigree chart, males are designated by
squares and females by circles. Shaded circles and squares
are afflicted individuals. A line between a square and a circle
represents a mating, and a double line represents a mating
between cousins. A vertical line going downward leads to the
children who are placed off a horizontal line if there are
several children. In this chart, the medical condition is
recessive and since cousins are more likely to carry the same
recessive genes, their children are more likely to show the
recessive phenotype.

carrier mates with another carrier, there is a 25 percent chance that any of their
children will show the condition. It is important to realize, though, that "chance
has no memory," thus, each child of these parents has a 25 percent chance
of having the trait. Therefore, it is possible that if a hybrid couple had four
children, each child might have the condition.

The pedigree chart shown here emphasizes the fact that a marriage of
close relatives (the double line indicates a marriage between first cousins) is apt
to bring out a recessive trait. Genetic diseases appear more frequently among
members of the same group, nationality, and/or race simply because members
of the same group, nationality, and/or race tend to marry one another. For

example, Tay-Sachs disease is seen more frequently among Jews; Cooley's anemia often occurs among Italians and Spaniards of Mediterranean descent; and sickle-cell anemia is frequently seen among blacks.

*Examples.* PKU (**phenylketonuria**) takes its name from the fact that phenylketone chemicals are present in the blood and urine of a person with this disease. Afflicted individuals (fig. 2.6) are unable to normally metabolize the common amino acid called phenylalanine. Therefore, the level of phenylalanine in the blood may rise to thirty times the normal amount. This abnormal metabolism leads to phenylketone chemicals in the urine. Unfortunately, the nervous system is affected most severely, and if the person goes untreated, severe mental retardation results.

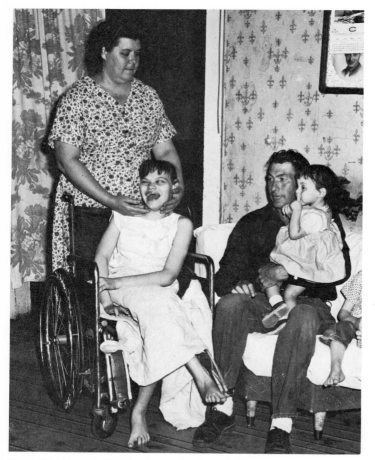

Figure 2.6   Person with PKU. (Source: March of Dimes Photo.)

Newborn babies are routinely tested at the hospital for PKU, and if diagnosed as having PKU, they are immediately placed on a diet low in phenylalanine. After about three years, this special diet may be discontinued even though the amount of phenylalanine then rises in the child's system. Evidently, large amounts of phenylalanine are only dangerous when the child's systems are still developing. This contention is borne out by the fact that women with PKU disease have children with abnormalities even when they mate with men who do not have the disease. The excess phenylalanine in the pregnant woman's blood can cross the placenta (p. 159) and affect the development of the fetus. To prevent this, these women can be placed on a diet low in phenylalanine.

**Tay Sachs** is a genetic disease that leads to deterioration and death a few years after birth. The victim is unable to break down a certain type of fat molecule that accumulates around nerve cells until they are destroyed.

A biochemical test can detect carriers of the recessive gene and can also be used to test fetal cells obtained by amniocentesis (p. 15). Tay Sachs disease is an example of more than sixty biochemical disorders that can now be detected prenatally as a result of the perfected technique of amniocentesis. Since there is no known cure for the disease, parents may elect to abort a fetus found to have Tay-Sachs disease.

PKU and Tay-Sachs may be used to illustrate the fact that the cost to society is minimized if genetic diseases are prevented and/or successfully treated. Figure 2.7 compares the cost of caring for a person with Tay-Sachs disease and PKU to that of screening and prevention. The cost of caring for a person with a genetic disease is usually borne by society because the individual rarely has adequate funds to meet these health care expenses.

Dominant Genetic Diseases

Figure 2.8 shows a pedigree chart for a dominant genetic disease.[5] A child that has the condition must have a parent with the condition unless, of course, a **mutation** (genetic change) has occurred (p. 70).

Usually an offspring afflicted with a dominant genetic disease has one hybrid parent and one pure recessive parent. Thus, the child had a 50 percent chance of getting the faulty gene or escaping it completely. Again, it must be remembered that chance has no memory, and since each child has the same genetic chance, it would be possible for several children in the same family to inherit a dominant genetic disease.

5. For other examples, see Appendix A.

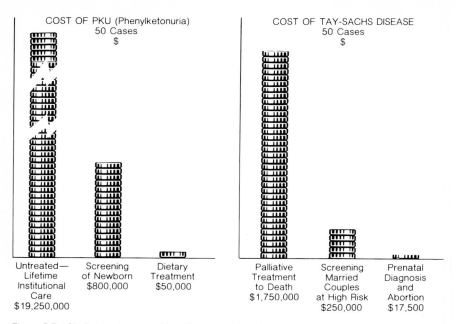

COST OF PKU (Phenylketonuria)
50 Cases
$

| Untreated— Lifetime Institutional Care $19,250,000 | Screening of Newborn $800,000 | Dietary Treatment $50,000 |

COST OF TAY-SACHS DISEASE
50 Cases
$

| Palliative Treatment to Death $1,750,000 | Screening Married Couples at High Risk $250,000 | Prenatal Diagnosis and Abortion $17,500 |

Figure 2.7   Studies to date reveal that the economic gain from screening and prevention can exceed by 10 to 20-fold the cost of caring medically for genetic disease victims. This calculation does not, of course, take into account the alleviation of anxiety and suffering by patients and their families. Illustrative cases have been made for PKU and Tay-Sachs disease.

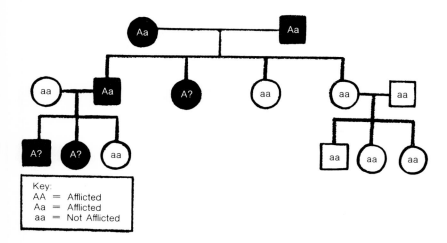

Key:
AA = Afflicted
Aa = Afflicted
aa = Not Afflicted

Figure 2.8   In a pedigree chart for a dominant characteristic, several individuals are more likely to show the phenotype.

**Chart 2.5**

Age Range at Onset for Genetic Diseases

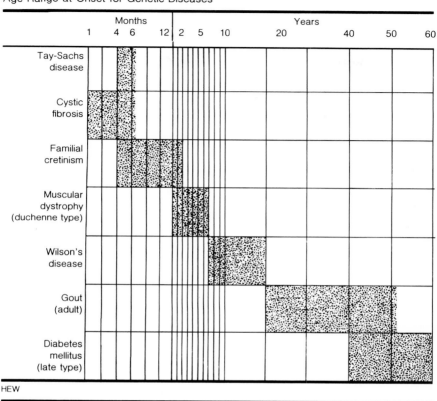

HEW

*Huntington's chorea.* Not all genetic diseases are immediately apparent at birth. Some, like Huntington's chorea, do not appear until midlife. Chart 2.5 indicates the time of life at which various other genetic diseases manifest their symptoms. Huntington's chorea is characterized by a progressive deterioration of the individual's nervous system that eventually leads to constant thrashing and writhing movements until insanity precedes death. The condition is difficult to diagnose, the progress of the disease is swift, and there is no known cure.

Estimates show that there are about 500 known cases of this disease in U.S. veterans' hospitals and that the cost of caring for these individuals is approximately $10 million a year. Since there is no known diagnostic test to detect this gene, the only prevention is for possible carriers not to have children.

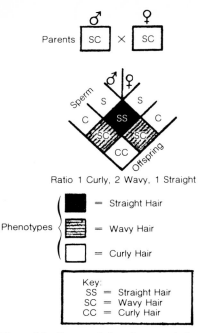

Ratio 1 Curly, 2 Wavy, 1 Straight

Phenotypes
= Straight Hair
= Wavy Hair
= Curly Hair

Key:
SS = Straight Hair
SC = Wavy Hair
CC = Curly Hair

Figure 2.9 Representation of a cross between two individuals with wavy hair. Neither curly nor straight hair is dominant; when these two genes are both present, the individual has wavy hair.

## Incomplete Dominance

It is possible for two genes to be partially expressed in which case both equally affect the phenotype.[6] For example, a union between a straight-haired person and a curly haired person produces children with wavy hair. In such cases, the most convenient symbolization is to assign a capital letter to both characteristics. Thus,

SS = straight hair
CC = curly hair
SC = wavy hair.

If two wavy haired individuals mate, any of the three phenotypes is possible. The chances for straight hair are 25 percent, the chances for wavy hair are 50 percent, and the chances for curly hair are 25 percent (fig. 2.9 ).

6. Sometimes called intermediate inheritance.

**Sickle-cell anemia** is an example of an incompletely dominant genetic disease in which:

AA  =  normal
SS  =  sickle-cell anemia
SA  =  sickle-cell trait.

The letter *S* stands for hemoglobin S and the letter *A* stands for hemoglobin A. Hemoglobin A is normal hemoglobin, the red respiratory pigment found in blood cells. Hemoglobin S molecules are relatively insoluble in water, and they tend to bind together to produce red cells that have a sicklelike shape (fig. 2.10).

A person with sickle-cell anemia (SS) has sickle-shaped cells that cannot pass easily along small blood vessels. The sickle-shaped cells either break down or they clog blood vessels. Thus, the individual suffers from poor circulation and anemia. Jaundice, episodic pain of the abdomen and joints, poor resistance to infection, and damage to internal organs are also symptoms of sickle-cell anemia. Few patients live beyond age forty.

Persons with the sickle-cell trait (SA) do not usually have any difficulties unless they are exposed to air that is low in oxygen. At such times, the cells become sickle-shaped with accompanying disturbances in circulation. Since 8 percent to 13 percent of Negroes are believed to have the sickling trait, the chances of a carrier mating with another carrier are considered to be higher than usual.

Sickle-cell anemia can be controlled by testing potential carriers testing and by fetal detection. An easily performed blood test can detect those with sickle-cell trait, and special centers have been established to quickly and conveniently test interested persons. Recently, a technique has been developed to detect the abnormal sickle-cell gene among chromosome fragments. Therefore, amni-

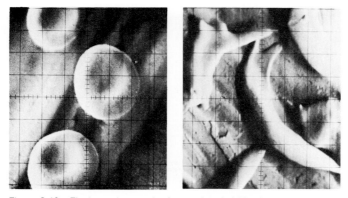

Figure 2.10  Electron micrograph of normal and sickle-shape blood cells. (Source: Phillips Electronic Instruments, Skokie, IL.)

ocentesis can now be used to determine if a baby will be born with sickle-cell anemia.

## Polygenic or Multifactor Inheritance

Some characteristics, such a height or skin color, seem to be controlled by more than one pair of genes. In these cases, it is possible to find a range of phenotypes (fig. 2.11) from one extreme to another, with most individuals falling somewhere in between. Considering the whole population, for example, there are few people who are very short and few who are very tall; most people are of average height.

Skin Color

When black persons mate with white persons, any resulting children are **mulatto**; but when two mulattoes mate, the skin color range of the offspring may vary considerably. It is possible to explain this range if you assume that two pairs of genes control skin color and that:

Black     =  AABB
Dark      =  AABb or aABB
Mulatto   =  AaBb or AAbb
            or aaBB
Light     =  Aabb or aabB
White     =  aabb.

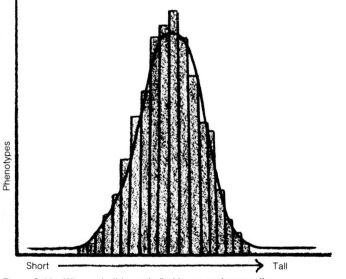

Figure 2.11   When a trait is controlled by several genes, the possible phenotypes differ by degree and the range of phenotypes in the population will assume a bell-shaped curve.

Notice that all dominant genes cause the person's skin to be black; any one recessive gene means that the person's skin is dark; any two recessive genes indicate that the person is a mulatto; any three recessive genes means the person's skin is light; all recessive genes make the person's skin white.

Sometimes rumors circulate that a woman who has light skin and is married to a white man has produced a black or dark-skinned child. However, this is genetically impossible by considering that a union between a light-skinned individual (Aabb) and a white-skinned individual (aabb) could at best give a child with only one dominant gene for skin color. Clearly, the darkest skin tone possible from this mating is light skin. Therefore, as long as this woman mates only with her husband, she cannot produce a dark-skinned or black child.

To carry the example even further, let us suppose, as illustrated in the pedigree chart (fig. 2.12), that this woman's grandmother was black. However,

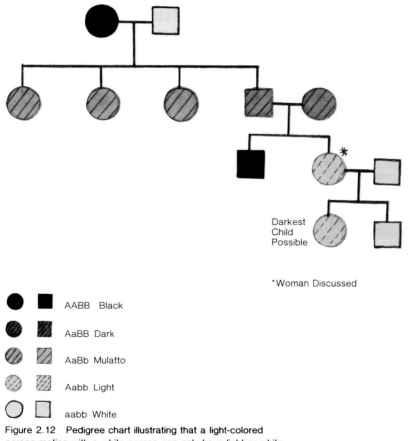

Darkest Child Possible

*Woman Discussed

| | | |
|---|---|---|
| ● | ■ | AABB  Black |
| ◕ | ◪ | AaBB  Dark |
| ◑ | ◨ | AaBb  Mulatto |
| ◔ | ◩ | Aabb  Light |
| ○ | □ | aabb  White |

Figure 2.12  Pedigree chart illustrating that a light-colored person mating with a white person can only have light or white children even if a sibling is black.

since her grandfather was white, all of the older couple's children were mulattoes. The woman under consideration is the result of a marriage between one of their mulatto children and another mulatto individual. Even if the woman had a black sibling (brother or sister), she still could not produce a black child. Each individual's genes are independent of any other person's genes!

Blood Types

The red cells of humans may have different types of chemicals, and blood is typed according to its red cell membrane chemical content. The most common designations for blood type are based on the presence of chemicals designated as A and B combined with the presence or absence of the substance called Rh factor.

Chart 2.6 lists possible blood types in terms of phenotype and genotype. The genotypes contain any two of three possible genes: A, B, or O. A person with type A blood can have either AA or AO genotype; a person with type B blood can have either BB or BO genotype. However, a person with AB type blood must have the genes AB and a person with Type O blood must have the genes OO.

From our study of genetics so far, it should come as no surprise that children can have a blood type different from that of either parent. For example, it is possible for individuals with blood type B to have an offspring that has blood type O:

Parents:        Type B × Type B
Child:          Type O

Obviously, these parents have the genotype BO.

However, it can also be seen that a parent with blood type AB cannot have a child that has type O blood:

Parents:        Type AB × Type OO
Children:       Type A or Type B

---

**Chart 2.6**
Frequency of Blood Types in the United States

| Phenotype | Genotype | Frequency in Caucasian Population (percent) | Frequency in Negro Population (percent) |
|-----------|----------|---------------------------------------------|------------------------------------------|
| Type AB | AB | 3 | 3.7 |
| Type B | BO, BB | 10 | 21 |
| Type A | AO, AA | 42 | 26 |
| Type 0 | OO | 45 | 49.3 |

---

Similarly, a person who has blood type O cannot have a child who has type AB. Such considerations can be used in cases of disputed paternity.

*Rh factor.*   Most Americans have blood type O+. The positive sign stands for the fact that their red cells contain a chemical called the Rh factor. The Rh factor is inherited as a simple dominant in which D = Rh factor and d = absence of the factor. Thus, it is possible for parents with Rh+ blood to have a child with Rh− blood if the parents are hybrids.

The Rh factor is of particular concern when the woman has Rh− (negative) blood and the man has Rh+ (positive) blood. In such a case, an offspring may, of course, have Rh+ blood. As illustrated in figure 2.13, the pregnant woman with Rh− blood may react to the blood cells of an Rh+ child by producing antibodies. This will occur just before or at the time of delivery when some of the child's blood cells can enter her system. If the woman becomes pregnant with another Rh+ child, these antibodies may cross the placenta and cause destruction of the unborn child's red cells, causing a condition called **erythroblastosis.**

The woman's body produced the antibodies because the Rh factor is an antigen for her.

*Antigens and antibodies.* **Antigens** are chemicals that the body recognizes as potentially harmful foreign substances. In response, the body produces **antibodies** to combine with antigens to reduce them to harmless complexes:

antigens + antibodies———➤harmless complex

● Rh Antigen    ↤ Rh Antibody

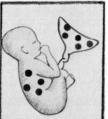 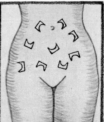 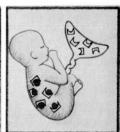

a. During Pregnancy      b. At Delivery      c. Months and Years Later      d. Subsequent Pregnancy

Figure 2.13   Diagrams describing the development of erythroblastosis. (a) Baby's red blood cells carry Rh antigen. (b) Some of these cells escape into the mother's circulatory system. (c) Mother begins to manufacture Rh antibodies. (d) During a subsequent pregnancy, mother's Rh antibodies cross placenta to destroy baby's red cells.

The production of antibodies is usually very beneficial because they normally protect us from serious contagious diseases such as those caused by bacteria or viruses. Unfortunately, in the case of the Rh factor, the woman's production of antibodies is undesirable and poses a serious threat to her unborn children.

*Erythroblastosis.*   Years ago, the only available treatment for erythroblastosis was an immediate blood transfusion for the newborn infant. Today, however, prevention of erythroblastosis is possible because women with Rh— blood can receive a Rho Gam injection immediately upon the birth of a child with Rh+ blood. The injection contains antibodies to the Rh factor. This may seem surprising until one realizes that a person receiving pre-formed antibodies is not likely to start self-production of that sort of antibodies. The theory behind the Rho Gam injection follows this principle. It is as follows:

The antibodies in the Rho Gam injection search out and destroy any Rh+ factors in the new mother's blood. Any unused antibodies soon disappear; and since the factors have been eliminated, the woman will never produce Rh antibodies herself. Therefore, any subsequent babies with Rh+ blood will be safe from attack.

*Combined blood type.*   For the combined blood type, it is necessary to consider the genes for A, B, O, and also those for the Rh factor. For example, a person who has blood type B+ could possibly have these genotypes: BBDD, or BODD, or BBDd, or BODd.

If a person with blood type BODd mates with a person having blood type AODd, what blood types might their children have? Simple examination shows that these blood types are possible: B+, B—, A+, A—, AB+, AB—, O+, O—, or all possible blood types.

## Polygenic Genetic Diseases

A number of serious genetic diseases, such as cleft lip or palate (fig. 2.14), club foot, congenital dislocation of the hip, and certain spine conditions, occur only when several different genes interact. Because a combination of genes brings about these conditions, it is difficult to predict the chances that any couple will have such a child.

However, if a couple is concerned about the birth of a child with a neural tube (nerve cord protected by vertebrae) defect, an analysis of the amniotic fluid, following amniocentesis, can reveal if there has been a leakage of neural tube substance into the fluid. If such a leakage has taken place, then it is known that the unborn child is not developing normally.

Amniocentesis can be used in several ways to detect fetal abnormalities; they are reviewed in chart 2.7.

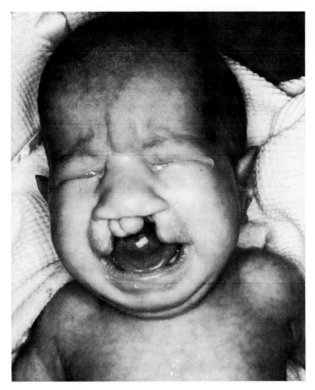

Figure 2.14   Child with cleft palate and hair lip. (Source: Dr. S. Schneider, Loma Linda University Medical School.)

## Chart 2.7
Indications for Amniocentesis

Chromosome studies on cultured amniotic fluid cells:
    Mother's age is greater than 35
    Previous child with Down's syndrome
    Family history or either parent is carrier for chromosomal disorder
    Determination of sex in X-linked disorders*

Biochemical studies on cultured amniotic fluid cells:
    Previous child with testable inborn error of metabolism**
    Parents are carriers for Tay-Sachs disease

Biochemical studies on amniotic fluid
    Previous child with neural tube defect

Gene studies on cultured amniotic fluid cells
    Parents are carriers for sickle-cell anemia
    Parents are carriers for $\alpha$-thalassemia***

*See pp. 49–52.
**See p. 66.
***See Appendix.

## Summary

Genes that are located within the chromosomes control the characteristics of an individual. A gene is assigned a capital letter if it is dominant and a lowercase letter if it is recessive. Each characteristic is usually controlled by a pair of genes; for example, the genotype Ee means that the individual has the phenotype free earlobes.

The use of Punnett Squares allows one to determine the phenotype ratio among the offspring because all possible sperm of a particular father are given an equal chance to fertilize all possible eggs of a particular mother. When a hybrid individual mates with another hybrid there is a 75 percent chance the offspring will show the dominant phenotype and a 25 percent chance the child will show the recessive phenotype. When a hybrid mates with a pure recessive, the offspring has a 50 percent chance of either phenotype.

Determination of inheritance is sometimes complicated by the fact that characteristics are controlled by incompletely dominant genes or by more than two genes, called polygenic inheritance. Blood type and skin color are examples of polygenic inheritance.

It is now known that many illnesses of humans are genetic in origin. Appendix A reviews common genetic diseases that are dominant, recessive, and polygenic. Sickle-cell anemia is incompletely dominant.

## Terms

| | |
|---|---|
| antibodies | genetic disease |
| antigens | genotype |
| autosomal dominant | hybrid |
| autosomal recessive | phenotype |
| carrier | polygenic |
| chance | pure dominant |
| erythroblastosis | pure recessive |

## Review

Problems in which the trait is dominant:

1. A woman hybrid for polydactyly is married to a normal man. What are the chances that her children will have six fingers and toes?

2. A young man's father has just been diagnosed as having Huntington's disease. What are the probable chances that the son will inherit this condition?

3. Black hair is dominant over blond hair. A woman with black hair whose father had blond hair has sexual relations and mates with a blond-haired man. What are the chances of this couple having a blond-haired child?

4. Your maternal grandmother Smith had Huntington's disease. Aunt Jane, your mother's sister, also had the disease. Your mother dies at age sixty-five with no signs of Huntington's disease. What are your chances of getting Huntington's disease?

5. Could a person who can curl her tongue have parents who cannot curl their tongues? Explain your answer.

Problems in which the trait is recessive:

6. Parents who do not have Tay-Sachs produce a child who has Tay-Sachs. What is the genotype of each parent? What are the chances each child will have Tay-Sachs?

7. One parent has galactosemia and the other is hybrid. What are the chances that their child will have galactosemia?

8. A child has cystic fibrosis. His parents are normal. What is the genotype of all persons mentioned?

Problems in which the trait is incompletely dominant:

9. What are the chances that a person pure for straight hair who is married to a person pure for curly hair will have children with wavy hair?

10. One parent has sickle-cell anemia and the other is perfectly normal. What are the phenotypes of their children?

11. A child has sickle-cell anemia but her parents do not. What is the genotype of each parent?

Problems in which the trait is controlled by several genes:

12. The genotype of a woman with type B blood is BO. The genotype of her husband is AO. What could be the genotypes and phenotypes of the children?

13. A man has type AB blood. What is his genotype? Could this man be the father of a child with type B blood? If not, why not? If so, what blood types could the child's mother have?

14. Baby Susan has type B blood. Both parents have type O blood. Are these the real parents?

15. A woman has type B+ blood and her husband-to-be has type A− blood. Assuming all possible genotypes, what blood types could their future children have? Could this marriage be one in which erythroblastosis might occur? Why or why not?

16. A woman with white skin has mulatto parents. Explain how this is possible. If this woman married a black man, what is the darkest skin color possible for their children? The lightest?

# 3

# Sex-Linked
# Inheritance

The sex chromosomes carry genes just as the autosomal chromosomes do. Most of these genes determine the sex of the individual, that is, whether the individual has testes or ovaries, but there are a few genes on the sex chromosomes that control traits unrelated to sex characteristics. They are called **sex-linked genes.**

Chart 3.1 lists some sex-linked recessive genetic diseases. These diseases are controlled by recessive genes on the X chromsome; the Y chromosome is blank for these genes.

It would be logical to suppose that sex-linked conditions are passed from father to son or from mother to daughter, but this is not the case. To understand

**Chart 3.1**
Sex-Linked Recessive Genetic Diseases

| Name | Symptoms | Defect | Comments |
|------|----------|--------|----------|
| Color blindness | Unable to see all colors | Receptors in eyes | Can lead normal life |
| Hemophilia | Blood does not clot | Factor VIII deficiency | Lifetime treatment; carriers can be detected; afflicted fetuses can be detected by blood test following fetoscopy |
| Muscular dystrophy | Muscle weakness | Muscle chemistry is faulty | Carriers can sometimes be detected; afflicted fetuses can be detected by blood test following fetoscopy |
| Lesch-Nyhan | Self-mutiliation; mental retardation | High blood level of uric acid | Carriers can be detected; afflicted fetuses can be detected following amniocentesis |
| Agamma-globulin-emia | Constant and severe infections | Unable to make antibodies | Some immunity genetic diseases are not sex-linked |

this, we will examine the sex-linked condition of color blindness. A proper key for color blindness would be:

$X^C$ = normal vision
$X^c$ = color blindness.

The letters are shown as superscripts of the X because these genes are carried on the X chromosome. Since the Y chromosome is blank for these genes, the following genotypes and phenotypes are possible for both sexes.

| *Females* | | | *Males* | | |
|---|---|---|---|---|---|
| $X^C X^C$ | = | perfectly normal | $X^C Y$ | = | normal |
| $X^C X^c$ | = | carrier | $X^c Y$ | = | color blind |
| $X^c X^c$ | = | color blind | | | |

Notice that because females have two X chromosomes, they may be carriers, but because males have only one X chromosome, they must show the recessive gene and be color blind. This is the reason that many more males than females have recessive sex-linked genetic diseases.

To determine the manner in which sex-linked recessive genetic diseases are inherited, we will consider three different matings in which the recessive gene for color blindness is involved.

1. When a female carrier mates with a normal male, the Punnett Square (fig. 3.1) shows that all female offspring will be normal even though they have a 50 percent chance of being a carrier. Males, on the other hand, have a 50 percent chance of being color blind because they have a 50 percent chance of inheriting the recessive gene from their mother. The inheritance from their father, which is always a Y, cannot offset this inheritance from their mother.

2. When a color-blind male mates with a normal female, the Punnett Square (fig. 3.2) shows that all children are normal even though all girls are carriers.

3. When a female carrier mates with a color-blind male (fig. 3.3), both male and female offspring have a 50 percent chance of being color blind. A boy is color blind when he receives the recessive gene from his mother. A girl is color blind when she receives the recessive gene from both parents. Therefore, for a girl to be color blind, her father must also be color blind. Since it is not likely that a carrier female will mate with a color-blind male, there are very few color-blind females.

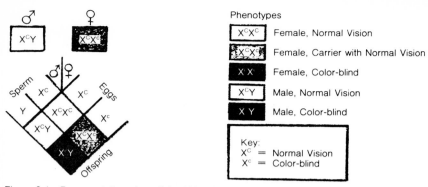

Phenotypes

| | |
|---|---|
| X$^C$X$^C$ | Female, Normal Vision |
| X$^C$X$^c$ | Female, Carrier with Normal Vision |
| X$^c$X$^c$ | Female, Color-blind |
| X$^C$Y | Male, Normal Vision |
| X$^c$Y | Male, Color-blind |

Key:
X$^C$ = Normal Vision
X$^c$ = Color-blind

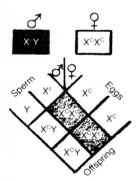

Figure 3.1   Representation of sex-linked inheritance. When the male parent is normal but the female parent is a carrier, daughters have a 50 percent chance of being a carrier and sons have a 50 percent chance of being color blind.

Figure 3.2   Representation of sex-linked inheritance when the male parent is color blind and the female parent is normal. Daughters will all be carriers and the sons will all be normal.

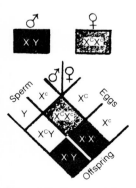

Figure 3.3   Representation of sex-linked inheritance when the male parent is color blind and the female parent is a carrier. Both sons and daughters have a 50 percent chance of being color blind.

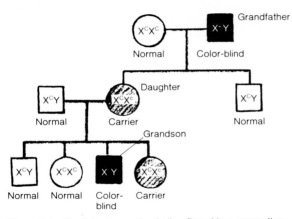

Figure 3.4   Sex-linked recessive traits often skip a generation and pass from grandfather to grandson by way of a carrier female. (After Mader, *Inquiry into Life,* 2d edition.)

*Pedigree chart.*   Figure 3.4 shows a possible family tree for a sex-linked recessive genetic disease. Notice that:

1. Only males have the condition; and
2. the condition skips a generation, going from grandfather through carrier daughter to grandson.

Both of these situations are common to sex-linked recessive genetic diseases. One feature of the family tree that is uncommon is that none of the males in the second generation escaped the condition even though each one had a 50 percent chance of inheriting either the recessive or dominant gene.

## Other Genetic Diseases

Hemophilia

**Hemophilia** is called the bleeder's disease because the afflicted person's blood is unable to clot. While hemophiliacs do bleed externally after an injury, they also suffer from internal bleeding, particularly around joints that are in frequent motion. Repeated joint bleeds can cause joint degeneration and muscle wasting.

The most common type of hemophilia—hemophilia A, or classic hemophilia—is due to the absence, or minimal presence, of a particular clotting factor called Factor VIII. When blood clots, twelve factors in the blood interact in a chain reaction to produce a blood clot; the lack of any one of these factors can cause hemophilia.

Years ago, a hemophiliac received blood plasma (the liquid portion of blood) to stop the bleeding. Today, concentrated Factor VIII is available and may be injected directly into the hemophiliac's system to stop the bleeding. In fact, concentrated Factor VIII is now available in a form that can be stored at home in the freezer. Some hemophiliacs routinely administer the factor so that the blood will clot automatically whenever necessary. Unfortunately, the cost of a single dose of AHF (antihemophiliac factor) concentrate can be as high as $100 or more. Often, this cost cannot be borne by the individual and outside financial assistance is necessary.

### Muscular Dystrophy

**Muscular dystrophy**, as the name implies, is characterized by the wasting away of muscles. The most common form, *Duchenne type*, is a sex-linked recessive disorder. Symptoms such as waddling gait, toe-walking, frequent falls, and difficulty in rising may appear as soon as the child starts to walk. Muscle weakness intensifies until the individual is confined to a wheel chair. Death usually occurs during the teenage years. At present, there is no specific therapy, but attempts are made to prolong activity by muscle-strengthening exercises, corrective surgical measures, and appropriate braces.

### Lesch-Nyhan Syndrome

Males who inherit this condition are mentally retarded and practice self-mutilation by chewing their lips and fingertips. The individual shows scars resulting from this practice (fig. 3.5) . Curiously, the metabolic abnormality consists of accumulation of uric acid in the blood.

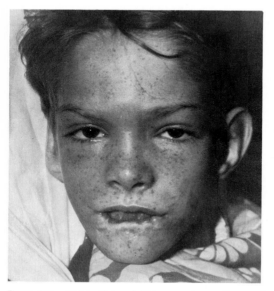

Figure 3.5    Child with Lesch-Nyhan syndrome. (Source: Dr. W.L. Nyhan.)

## Agammaglobulinemia

Persons who have **agammaglobulinemia** (fig. 3.6) are unable to manufacture antibodies and, therefore, are susceptible to repeated infections. To prevent this occurrence, they sometimes must spend their lives in a protective sterile bubble or a protective suit of some sort.

Normally, the *lymphocytes,* a type of white blood cell, produce antibodies that fight infection. Since a person with agammaglobulinemia is unable to make antibodies, this natural protection against infection is an impossibility.

## Prevention

The symptoms of these sex-linked genetic recessive disorders are extremely disabling and require that the individual receive a great deal of care. Therefore, women who wish to have children and suspect that they might be carriers may undergo tests to determine if indeed they are carriers.

For carrier women, amniocentesis can reveal if the unborn child is a male. Once it has been determined that the woman is carrying a male, a technique

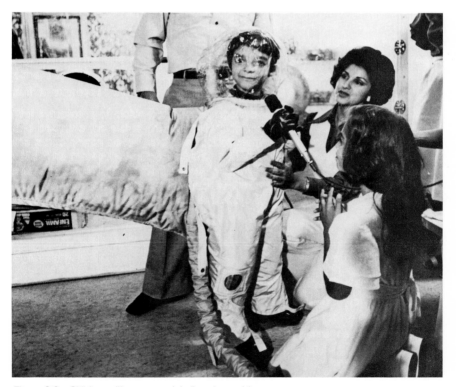

Figure 3.6   Children with agammaglobulinemia must be protected from infections. (Source: NASA.)

called fetoscopy (insertion of an optical device into the uterus by way of the abdominal wall) can be used to locate one of baby's blood vessels in the placenta (p. 159). Using an extremely narrow needle, a few drops of the baby's blood can be removed and analyzed for Factor VIII in the case of hemophilia and for a chemical called CPK (creatine phosphokinase) if muscular dystrophy is suspected. Should the fetus test positive for these conditions, an abortion may be performed.

## Sex-Limited Traits

Sex-limited traits are characteristics that often appear in one sex but only rarely appear in the other. It's believed that these traits are governed by genes that are turned on or off by hormones. For example, the secondary sex characterisitics such as the beard of a male and the breasts of a female probably are indirectly controlled by hormone balance.

Baldness (fig. 3.7) is believed to be caused by the male sex hormone, testosterone, because males who take the hormone to increase masculinity begin to lose their hair. A more detailed explanation has been suggested by

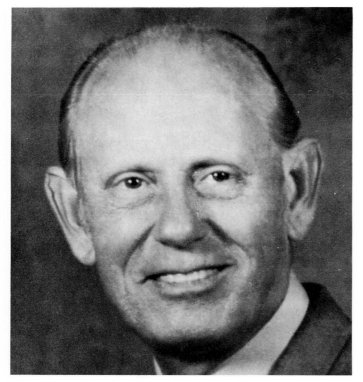

Figure 3.7    Baldness is a sex-influenced characteristic.
(Source: Dr. A.M. Winchester.)

some investigators. It has been reasoned that due to the effect of hormones, males require only one gene for the trait to appear, whereas females require two genes. In other words, the gene acts as a dominant in males but as a recessive in females. This means that males born to a bald father and a mother with hair *at best* would have a 50 percent chance of going bald. Females born to a bald father and a mother with hair at *worst* would have a 25 percent chance of going bald.

## Summary

Sex-linked genes are located on the X chromosome. Since the Y chromosome does not carry these genes, only the gene received from the mother determines the phenotype in males. This means that males are more apt to display a trait controlled by a sex-linked recessive gene. It also indicates that if a female does have the phenotype, then her father must also have it. Usually sex-linked traits skip a generation and go from maternal grandfather to grandson.

Genetic diseases are sometimes sex linked. Those of particular interest are listed in Appendix A.

## Terms

Sex-limited gene
Sex-linked inheritance
Sex-linked recessive gene

## Review

1. A boy has agammaglobulinemia. What are the genotypes of the parents, who appear to be normal?
2. A woman is color blind and her spouse is normal. If they produce a son and a daughter, which child will be color blind?
3. If a female who carries a sex-linked gene has sexual relations and mates with a normal man, what are the chances that male children will have the condition? That female children will have the condition?
4. A girl has hemophilia. What is the genotype of her father? Of her mother, who appears to be normal?
5. What is the genotype of a man who is color blind and has a continuous hairline? If this man mates with a woman who is pure dominant for vision and widow's peak, what will the children be like?

Pedigree Charts
6. Are the traits (shaded circles and squares) below autosomal dominant, autosomal recessive, or sex-linked recessive?

a.

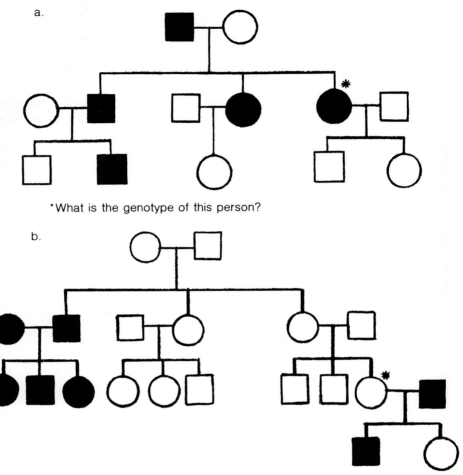

*What is the genotype of this person?

b.

*What is the genotype of this person?

C.

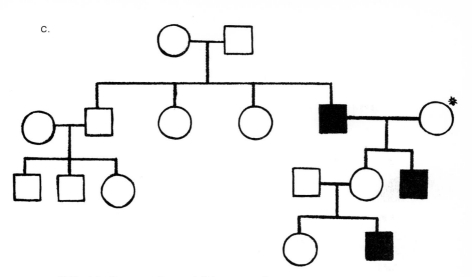

*What is the genotype of this person?

# 4

# Biochemical Genetics

Our approach to genetics thus far has been to consider the genes as particulate units of a chromosome. In contrast, **biochemical genetics** takes up the chemical nature of the gene and the biochemical function of genes in the cell.

DNA

Genes are made up of a chemical called DNA. This means that DNA is the *genetic material* and that chromosomes contain DNA. In fact, DNA is found principally in the nucleus of a cell (fig. 1.1).

DNA is a type of nucleic acid, and like all nucleic acids, it is formed by the sequential joining of smaller molecules called **nucleotides.** Nucleotides, in turn, are composed of three molecules—a **base**, a **phosphate**, and a **sugar**. The sugar in DNA is deoxyribose, which accounts for the chemical's name, *deoxyribonucleic acid.* There are four nucleotides (fig. 4.1) in DNA because there are four bases: Adenine **(A)**, Thymine **(T)**, Cytosine **(C)**, and Guanine **(G)**.

```
Phosphate
  |
Sugar ——— Adenine
```

```
Phosphate
  |
Sugar ——— Thymine
```

```
Phosphate
  |
Sugar ———Cytosine
```

```
Phosphate
  |
Sugar ———Guanine
```

Figure 4.1   The four nucleotides in DNA each contains phosphoric acid (phosphate); the sugar, deoxyribose, and a base which may be either Adenine (A), Thymine (T), Cytosine (C), or Guanine (G).

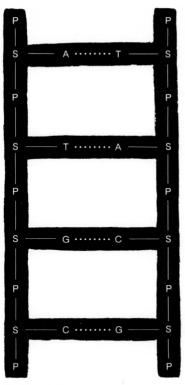

P = Phosphate
S = Sugar = Deoxyribose
A, T, G, C = Bases

Figure 4.2 Ladder structure of DNA is caused by the fact that the sugar and phosphate molecules form a backbone while the bases pair complementarily. Adenine pairs with Thymine and Guanine pairs with Cytosine, and vice versa.

*Ladder structure.* When nucleotides join together, the sugar and the phosphate molecules become a **backbone** and the bases project to the side (fig. 4.2). In DNA, there are two such chains of nucleotides held together by weak bonds between the bases; consequently, DNA is **double-stranded**. Each base is bonded to another particular base, called its **complementary base**—adenine (A) is always paired with thymine (T), and cytosine (C) is always paired with guanine (G). The reverse of these statements is, of course, also true. The dotted lines in figure 4.2 portray the weak bonds between the bases. The structure of DNA is said to resemble a *ladder* (fig. 4.3a) because the sugar-phosphate molecules appear to make up the sides of a ladder and the bases seem to make the steps. The ladder structure of DNA twists to form a spiral staircase called a **double helix** (fig. 4.3b). DNA is most often represented in this double helix form.

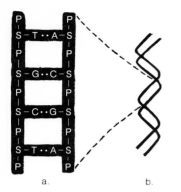

a.                    b.

Figure 4.3   The ladder structure twists to form a double helix.
A chromatid (p. 7) is one complete double helix.

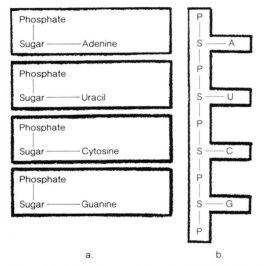

a.                              b.

Figure 4.4   (a) The four nucleotides in RNA each has a
phosphate molecule; the sugar, ribose, and a base which may
be either Adenine (A), Uracil (U), Cytosine (C), or Guanine (G).
(b) RNA is single-stranded. The sugar and phosphate
molecules join to form a backbone and the bases project to
the side.

**Chart 4.1**
DNA-RNA Similarities

Both are nucleic acids
Both are composed of nucleotides
Both have a sugar-phosphate backbone
Both have four different type bases

**Chart 4.2**
DNA-RNA Differences

| DNA | RNA |
| --- | --- |
| Found in nucleus | Found in nucleus and cytoplasm |
| The genetic material | Helper to DNA |
| Sugar is deoxyribose | Sugar is ribose |
| Bases are A, T, C, G | Bases are A, U, C, G |
| Double-stranded | Single-stranded |

RNA

RNA is nucleic acid that is made up of nucleotides containing the sugar ribose. This sugar accounts for its scientific name, *ribonucleic acid*. The nucleotides making up RNA also have four possible bases: Adenine (A), Uracil (U), Cytosine (C), and Guanine (G) (fig. 4.4). RNA, unlike DNA, is always single-stranded. Similarities and differences between these two nucleic acid molecules are given in charts 4.1 and 4.2.

Functions of DNA

*Duplication.* In between cell divisions, the daughter chromosomes must **replicate**, or **duplicate**, before cell division can occur again. Actually, when chromosomes duplicate, DNA is making a copy of itself. Duplication has been found to require the following steps:

1. The two strands that make up DNA become "unzipped" (i.e., the weak bonds between the paired bases break).
2. New complementary nucleotides, always present in the nucleus,[1] move into place beside each old strand by the process of base pairing.
3. These new complementary nucleotides become joined together.
4. When the process is finished, two complete DNA molecules are present, identical to each other and to the original molecule.

1. The food we eat is digested to molecules such as nucleotides and amino acids which are carried in the bloodstream to the cells.

Each new double helix (fig. 4.5) is composed of an old and a new strand. The new strand beside each old one is not exactly like the old strand; rather, each new strand is *complementary* to the old strand. Because of this, it is said that each strand of DNA serves as a **template**, or mold, for the production of its complementary strand. The entire duplication process is called **semi-conservative** because old strands are always paired with new strands.

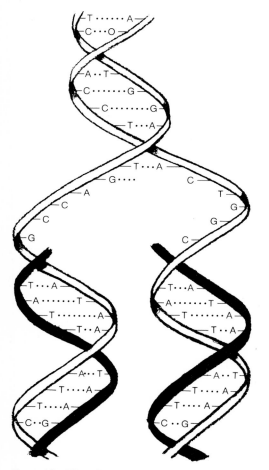

Figure 4.5   When DNA duplicates, the molecule unzips and each strand serves as a template for a complementary strand. (After Mader, *Inquiry into Life,* 2d edition.)

*Protein synthesis.* DNA directs the synthesis, or production, of proteins. Proteins are found in all cells. The protein hemoglobin is responsible for the red color of red blood cells. The antibodies, already mentioned on page 41, are proteins and there are other proteins in the blood as well. Muscle cells have much protein, giving them substance and their ability to contract.

Certain proteins are **enzymes** that speed up chemical reactions in cells. Actually, cells are chemical factories in which reactions are constantly and quickly occurring even though the body has a relatively low temperature. Reactions occur quickly in cells because of the presence of enzymes.

The reactions in cells form chemical or **metabolic pathways**. One such pathway could be represented as follows:

$$A \xrightarrow{\ 1\ } B \xrightarrow{\ 2\ } C \xrightarrow{\ 3\ } D \xrightarrow{\ 4\ } E$$

In this pathway the letters are molecules and the numbers are enzymes: Molecule *A* becomes molecule *B* and enzyme 1 speeds up the reaction; molecule *B* becomes molecule *C* and enzyme 2 speeds up the reaction, and so forth. Notice that each reaction in the pathway has its own enzyme; enzyme 1 can only convert *A* to *B*; enzyme 2 can only convert *B* to *C*; and so forth. For this reason, enzymes are said to be **specific**.

Structure.  **Proteins** are very large chemical molecules composed of individual units called **amino acids**. An amino acid joined to an amino acid joined to an amino acid, ad infinitum, results in a protein. There are twenty different common amino acids found in proteins. Proteins differ one from the other because the order of the amino acids differs (fig. 4.6). When DNA directs protein synthesis, it directs the order of the amino acids in a particular protein. It can do this because every three bases in *DNA* code (chart 4.3), or stand, for one amino acid. Thus, it is said that DNA contains a **triplet code**.

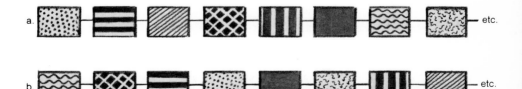

Figure 4.6  Proteins are made up of amino acid molecules (represented here by rectangles) linked together. There are twenty different amino acids and their sequence differs from one protein (a) to another (b).

## Chart 4.3

DNA Code and mRNA Codon

| DNA Code | mRNA Codon | tRNA Anticodon | Amino Acids (designated by patterns) |
|---|---|---|---|
| AAA | UUU | AAA | |
| ACC | UGG | ACC | |
| AAC | UUG | AAC | |
| TAC | AUG | UAU | |

Transcription.   Referring again to the structure of the cell (fig. 1.1), we mentioned previously that *DNA* is found in the nucleus. Protein synthesis occurs at the **ribosomes**, which are located in the cytoplasm or on a membrane called the *endoplasmic reticulum.* Therefore, it is obvious that there must be some inter-mediary way of getting the DNA message, or code, to the ribosomes. A molecule called *mRNA* (**messenger RNA**) takes the message from the DNA in the nucleus to the ribosome in the cytoplasm. Just as DNA can serve as a template for the production of itself, it can also serve as a template for the production of mRNA. During this process called **transcription**, RNA nucleotides complementary to one DNA strand join. The mRNA that results (fig. 4.7) has a sequence of bases complementary to those of DNA. While DNA contains a code in which every three bases stand for one amino acid, mRNA contains **codons**, each of which is made up of three bases that also stand for an amino acid (see chart 4.3). After formation, mRNA moves to the cytoplasm where it becomes attached to the ribosomes. (Ribosomes themselves are made of RNA called rRNA [ribosomal RNA].)

Translation.   The next step leading to protein synthesis is called **translation** because the order of the condons in mRNA is translated into a particular order of amino acids in a protein. For this to happen, free (or unattached) amino acids in the cytoplasm [2] must move to the vicinity of the ribosomes. To accomplish this transfer, another type of RNA called **transfer RNA** (*tRNA*) brings the amino acids to the ribosomes. There is a separate tRNA for every amino acid; therefore,

2. See footnote, p. 59.

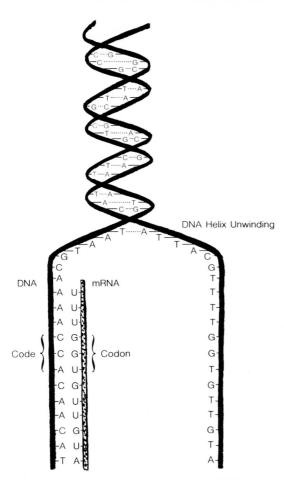

Figure 4.7 During transcription, one strand of DNA serves as a template for the production of mRNA; the completed mRNA strand is complementary to the DNA strand.

there are twenty different tRNA molecules. Each tRNA has three particular nucleotides whose bases make up an **anticodon** (fig. 4.8). Each anticodon is complementary to a particular codon.

As the ribosomes move along the mRNA, a particular codon becomes prominent. The tRNA, which has the complementary anticodon at one end and the appropriate amino acid at the other, moves into place. Thus, the sequence of the codons dictates the sequence of the tRNA molecules and this, in turn, dictates the order of the amino acids in a protein. By this indirect process, the

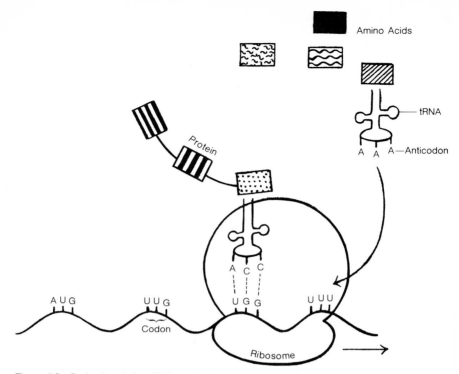

Figure 4.8 During translation, tRNA molecules bring amino acids to the ribosomes in the order dictated by the mRNA codons.

DNA code eventually controls the sequence of amino acids in proteins and thus in enzymes.

The entire transcription-translation sequence is diagrammed in figure 4.9.

*Steps in protein synthesis.* It is now possible to list the steps involved in protein synthesis. Chart 4.4 also contains pertinent information.

1. DNA, which remains in the nucleus, contains a series of bases that serve as a *triplet code* (a sequence of three bases).

2. One strand of DNA serves as a template for the formation of messenger RNA (mRNA) that contains triplet codons (sequences of three complementary bases).

3. Messenger RNA goes into the cytoplasm and becomes associated with the *ribosomes* that are composed of ribosomal RNA (rRNA).

4. Transfer RNA (tRNA) molecules, each of which is bonded to a particular amino acid, have *anticodons* that pair complementarily to the codons in mRNA.

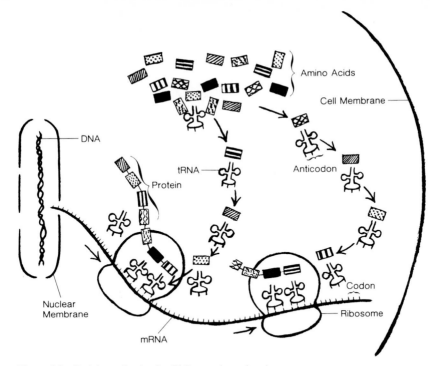

Figure 4.9  Protein synthesis. A mRNA complementary to a
DNA strand moves from the nucleus to the ribosomes. As the
ribosomes move along the mRNA, tRNA molecules transfer
amino acids in the order originally dictated by the DNA code
and immediately dictated by the mRNA codons. (Source: Vivian
M. Null, *Study Guide to Accompany Curtis: Invitation to
Biology*, 2d edition, Worth Publishers, New York, 1977.)

**Chart 4.4**
Steps in Protein Synthesis

| Name of Molecule | Special Significance | Definition |
| --- | --- | --- |
| DNA | Code | Sequence of bases in threes |
| mRNA | Codon | Complementary sequence of bases in threes |
| tRNA | Anticodon | Sequence of three bases complementary to codon |
| Amino acids | Building blocks | Transported to ribosomes by tRNAs |
| Protein | Enzymes | Amino acids joined in a predetermined order |

5. Transfer RNA molecules, along with their amino acids, come to the ribosomes in the order dicated by mRNA, and in this way *amino acids* become ordered in a particular sequence.

6. As the amino acid chain lengthens, a *specific* protein begins to form.

7. The transfer RNA molecules repeat the process of transporting amino acids to the ribosomes until the protein molecule is completed.

Metabolic Diseases

Many genetic diseases are now known to be the result of the inheritance of a faulty DNA code. Such a DNA contains a code for an inappropriate sequence of amino acids in an enzyme and the enzyme is thus nonfunctional. For example, one particular metabolic pathway in cells is:

A (phenylalanine)——$\xrightarrow{2}$——>B (tyrosine)——$\xrightarrow{3}$——>C (melanin)

$\downarrow$ 4

D (phenylketone).

If a person inherits a faulty code for enzyme 2 above, the genetic disease PKU (phenylketonuria) results (p. 32). Such a person is unable to convert the chemical phenylalanine (A) to tyrosine (B). Phenylalanine builds up in the system and eventually appears in the urine as phenylketone. The excess phenylalanine causes mental retardation and the other symptoms of PKU.

In this same pathway, if a person inherits a faulty code for enzyme 3, then tyrosine cannot be converted to melanin and the individual is an albino (fig. 4.10).

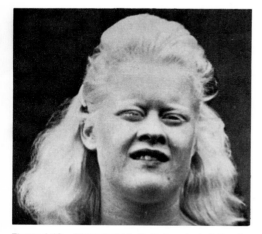

Figure 4.10 Albino individuals lack melanin (skin pigment) because they inherited a gene that codes improperly for an enzyme. (Source: A.M. Winchester.)

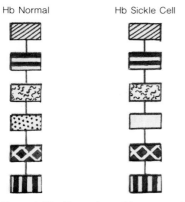

Hb Normal          Hb Sickle Cell

Figure 4.11    The amino acid sequence in sickle-cell
hemoglobin differs from normal hemoglobin by only one amino
acid. This illustrates that genes determine amino acid
sequences.

*Sickle-cell anemia.*    Since DNA codes for all proteins, genetic defects can involve proteins that are not enzymes. For example, sickle-cell anemia is caused by the inheritance of a faulty code for hemoglobin. It is now known that there is only one amino acid change between normal hemoglobin and sickle-cell hemoglobin (fig. 4.11). This one amino acid change causes the hemoglobin molecules to adhere to one another in such a way that the cells take on a sickle shape. One author expresses the situation in the following way:

The symptoms of sickle-cell anemia occur because the cells die off quickly and because the sickle-shaped cells clog the blood vessels. The cells have the sickle shape because of the rodlike clumping of molecules within the cells. The molecules clump that way because in one tiny spot a chemical attaches on differently than it does in normal red blood cell molecules. The tiny chemical (an amino acid) attaches that way because of the genes that were inherited from the person's ancestors.[3]

## Summary

Chromosomes are composed of DNA, a double-stranded molecule that contains a triplet code utilizing four bases: A, T, C, G. By means of complementary base pairing DNA serves as a template for its own replication and for the transcription of messenger RNA, a single-stranded nucleic acid that contains codons utilizing the four bases A, U, C, G.

3.  S. M. Linde, *Sickle Cell* (New York: Pavilion Publishing Co.,
    520 E. 77th St., New York, N.Y., 1972).

Messenger RNA moves from the nucleus to the cytoplasm where ribosomes composed of ribosomal RNA aid in the process of translation. Transfer RNA molecules carry amino acid molecules to the ribosomes where they become linked together in the order predetermined by the DNA code. The resulting protein molecules have various functions in cells but are notably enzymes involved in a metabolic pathway.

Genetic diseases are often inborn errors of metabolism because the inheritance of a faulty genetic code leads to a defective enzyme. Sickle-cell anemia, on the other hand, is caused by the inheritance of a faulty code for hemoglobin, a component of red cells.

---

## Terms

| | |
|---|---|
| amino acid | nucleic acid |
| bases | nucleotide |
| complementary base pairing | protein |
| DNA | protein synthesis |
| double helix | RNA |
| duplication | semiconservative |
| enzyme | strand |
| ladder structure | transcription |
| metabolic disease | translation |

---

## Review

1. Describe the structure of DNA.
2. How does DNA duplicate itself? When does it duplicate itself?
3. How does DNA structure differ from RNA structure?
4. Define nucleotide, nucleic acid, base, sugar, phosphate.
5. Describe the structure of proteins. How many different types of amino acids are there?
6. Compare code to codon to anticodon. What does the term complementary base pairing mean?
7. If ATCGITACCG were in DNA, what would the code be? The codons? The anticodons?
8. What role do ribosomes play in protein synthesis?
9. What do the terms mRNA, rRNA, and tRNA mean? What does each of these do in protein synthesis?
10. Locate the molecules in number 9 in the cell.

11. Explain protein synthesis, starting with DNA and finishing with the protein. Be sure to mention code, codon, anticodon, mRNA, tRNA, amino acids, and ribosomes in your answer.

12. What's wrong with someone who has PKU? Describe in terms of faulty code and faulty enzyme.

13. What's wrong with someone who has sickle-cell anemia? Describe in terms of faulty code and faulty hemoglobin.

# 5

# Modern Genetic Concerns

The basic structure and function of DNA, the genetic material, are now known; therefore, the possibility of eventually being able to directly control the genotype does exist. In the meantime, responsible scientists wish to prevent mutation, or gene changes, due to adverse environmental influences; to learn more about protein synthesis, particularly how it is controlled; and to develop ways to cure genetic diseases.

Mutations

Permanent changes in the DNA code are called **mutations**. Mutations may be either germinal or somatic.

*Germinal mutations.* A *germinal mutation* occurs whan a genetic change takes place during the maturation of gametes. Germinal mutations are recognized when the offspring shows a genetic disease. Chart 5.1 gives estimations for the number of times per 1 million gametes a certain gene change results in a particular genetic disease. For example, it is believed that 10 to 70 times per 1 million gametes there is a gene change such that the offspring has **Acondroplastic dwarfism** characterized by disproportionate shortening of the arms and legs. The mutation rate given here is assumed to be the natural mutation rate. In other words, a certain number of mutations occur spontaneously and are due to no particular cause.

*Somatic mutations.* A *somatic mutation* is one that affects only the individual's body cells. We are most familiar with somatic mutations that accompany cancer. When cancer develops, a mother cell produces cancerous daughter cells that divide to produce more cancerous cells. Cancer is apparent when cells grow in a haphazard and uncontrolled manner.

Although geminal and somatic mutations occur spontaneously (due to no known cause), the rate of mutation can be increased by environmental factors. Agents that cause mutations are called **mutagens.**

**Chart 5.1**

Estimates of Human Mutation Rates

| Trait | Mutations Per Million Gametes Per Generation |
|---|---|
| Retinoblastoma<br>Dominant; an eye tumor | 15–23 |
| Juvenile amaurotic idiocy<br>Recessive; blindness, paralysis, mental deficiency,<br>death, onset at about six years of age; common in<br>Scandinavia | 38 |
| Infantile amaurotic idiocy (Tay-Sachs disease)<br>Recessive; symptoms as above, but onset around<br>two years of age; common in Jews | 11 |
| Microcephaly<br>Recessive; abnormally small skull | 49 |
| Achondroplastic dwarfism<br>Dominant | 10–70 |
| Hemophilia<br>Sex-linked | 25–32 |
| Muscular dystrophy<br>Sex-linked | 43–100 |
| Albinism<br>Recessive | 28 |
| Aniridia<br>Dominant; absence of iris | 5 |
| Deaf-mutism<br>Several loci | 450 |
| Low-grade mental defect<br>Many loci | 1,500 |
| All loci causing death before early adulthood | 40,000 |

Adapted from *Heredity, Evolution and Society*, second edition, by I. Michael Lerner and William J. Libby. W.H. Freeman and Company. Copyright © 1976.

*Environmental mutagens.* Any environmental factor that increases the chances of a mutation is a mutagen. When a mutagen leads to an increase in the incidence of cancer, it is called a **carcinogen.** There are two broad categories of mutagens: *chemical mutagens* and *radiation*.

Suspected chemical mutagens range from food additives and hallucinogenic drugs (fig. 5.1) to pesticides and certain chemicals used in manufacturing. The Food and Drug Administration (FDA) is well known for taking food additives such as the chemical sweeteners off the market. These additives have been shown to be carcinogenic in laboratory animals, usually mice. In these experiments, large quantities of the chemical in question were fed to animals and the deleterious effects are noted. Since experimental consumption far exceeds normal

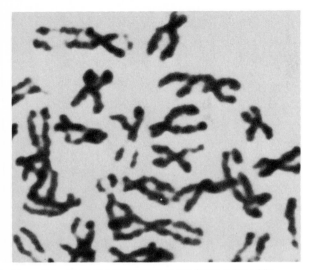

Figure 5.1   Damaged chromosomes are found in the white cells of individuals who have used LSD. (Source: Courtesy of J. Egozcue, Universidad Autónoma de Barcelona.)

human consumption, it is almost impossible to judge whether the results of these experiments can be corrrectly applied to humans. The federal law, however, is conservative and any chemical known to have carcinogenic effects cannot be added to food or used in food packaging.

The pesticides DDT, dieldrin, and aldrin have been shown to be mutagenic, and their use in the United States is now banned or restricted by the government. In regard to industrial chemicals such as vinyl chloride, the government tests the emission rate or atmospheric content in the vicinity of a chemical factory and if the level is judged to be unsafe, the plant in question may be shut down. The workers themselves are protected from dangerous chemicals by the Occupational Safety and Hazards Act (OSHA). However, accidents that endanger the health of nearby residents do occasionally occur.

Sometimes the government requires only that a warning label be placed on a consumer product containing carcinogens. Recently, it has been shown that hair dyes containing a chemical known as 2,4-DAS cause tumors when eaten in large quantities by mice, and the FDA has proposed that these products carry warning labels. Cigarette packs, of course, have such labels, and it is generally accepted that cigarette smoking is a frequent cause of lung cancer. The somatic changes leading to this condition are depicted in figure 5.2.

Like certain chemicals, radiation is also mutagenic. Humans are exposed to two types of radiation: natural and manmade (chart 5.2). *Radiation* occurs

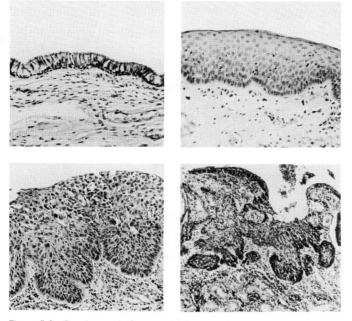

Figure 5.2  Development of cancer (a) Increase in number of cells in general. (b) Increase in number of cells with atypical nuclei. (c) Carcinoma in situ. (d) Cancer cells in the process of spreading to new locations. (Source: Photomicrographs by Oscar Auerbach, M.D., Veterans Administration Hospital, East Orange, N.J.)

## Chart 5.2

Approximate Average Doses of Ionizing Radiation from Various Sources to the Gonads of the General Population

| Source of Radiation | Average Dose Per Year (mrem) | Average Dose Per 30 Years (rems)[*] |
|---|---|---|
| Natural: | | |
| Cosmic radiation | 30 | 0.90 |
| Earth radiation | 50 | 1.50 |
| Ingested natural radiation | 20 | 0.60 |
| Man-made; | | |
| Medical radiology | 35 | 1.05 |
| Radioactive fallout | 1 | 0.03 |
| Nuclear power industry | 1 | 0.03 |
| Occupational and miscellaneous | 2 | 0.06 |
| Total | 139 | 4.17 |

[*]From Table 2 of the BEIR (Advisory Committee on the Biological Effects of Ionizing Radiations), 1972, p. 19.

in the form of electromagnetic radiation and radioactive elements. Short electromagnetic waves, such as x rays and gamma rays, and radiation from radioactive elements, such as Iodine 131 and Plutonium 210, have the ability to penetrate tissues and cause both somatic and germinal mutations. Longer electromagnetic waves, such as ultraviolet waves and microwaves, do not cause germinal mutations, but they can cause skin cancer and/or burns in susceptible individuals.

Natural radiation is radiation that originates from outer space and from radioactive elements in the ground and atmosphere. This so-called "background" radiation does contribute to the incidence of cancer and genetic disease in humans, but another source contributes more. Man-made radiation is believed to be an even more important contributor to occurrences of cancer and genetic diseases in humans. Many persons express concern about radiation exposure due to the nuclear power industry, but actually medical diagnostic radiation accounts for at least 90 percent of human exposure to man-made radiation (fig. 5.3). And the incidence of cancer has been shown to be higher in groups of individuals who have been exposed to x-ray treatment. For example, children who received x-ray treatment for swollen tonsils and adenoids during the 1930s, 1940s, and 1950s are now showing a high incidence of thyroid cancer, and deaths from leukemia are higher among children who were exposed to radiation while in the womb before birth. It has even been suggested that methods used to detect cancer of the breast could actually be causing cancer to develop.

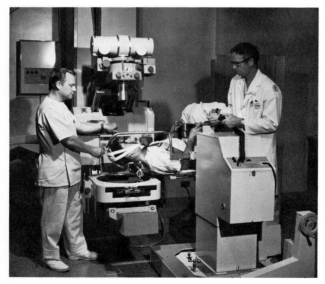

Figure 5.3   Patient undergoing X-ray diagnosis. (Source: American College of Radiology.)

Inheritance

Strong doses of radiation will kill cells. Because of this, radiation is used in the treatment of cancer. Even though the radiation is directed toward the malignant tissue, cancer patients often develop radiation sickness with accompanying nausea, diarrhea, headache, and malaise.

The current policy of the Environmental Protection Agency (EPA) is to assume that any level of radiation is potentially dangerous and that the danger increases as the radiation dose increases. Small doses of radiation over a long period of time are not as dangerous as large doses within a short period. Even so, it would be possible to achieve a reduction of radiation exposure of the United States population if (1) repetitive x-ray treatments were eliminated, (2) lead aprons were used to shield areas of the body, especially the pelvis, and (3) radiation equipment, techniques, and the training of personnel were improved.

Chemical mutagens and radiation are just two possible causes for the occurrence of cancer in humans. Some scientists believe that cancer is also caused by viral infections, hormonal imbalance, and failure of the immune system. Regardless of the cause, there does seem to be a genetic component to the development of cancer. Some investigators believe that cancer could be controlled by controlling environmental factors and others believe that it might eventually be possible to genetically prevent the occurence of cancer. The latter possibility is dependent in part on the success of the research work discussed as follows.

## Modern Genetic Research

Both *in vitro* and *in vivo* experiments are commonplace in genetic research. **In vitro** means that cell parts and molecules are studied in a test tube, while **in vivo** means that living organisms participate in the experiment. All sorts of experiments have been done in which cell parts, such as ribosomes and chromosomes, have been extracted from cells so that their structure and function can be studied in the test tube. As far as genes are concerned, the following processes have been done in whole or in part for a few genes (mostly animal genes but some are human genes):

1. Isolation of the gene, i.e., removal of just a particular portion of DNA (fig. 5.4) from a cell.
2. Determination of the sequence of nucleotides of the gene.
3. Manufacture of a man-made gene, i.e., joining nucleotides together in the proper sequence.
4. Placement of an isolated or man-made gene in another cell where it undergoes replication.
5. Placement of an isolated or man-made gene in another cell where it replicates and directs protein synthesis.

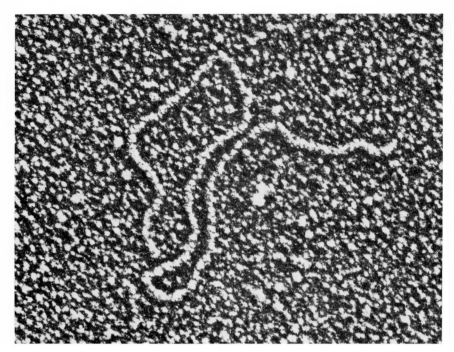

Figure 5.4   Electron micrograph of a piece of DNA. It is actually .000055 inches long. (Source: HEW)

In regard to 4 and 5, genes have most often been placed in the bacterium *E. coli*, and these experiments have come to be known as recombinant DNA experiments.

Recombinant DNA or Plasmid Experiments

Certain bacteria, such as *E. coli*, contain extrachromosomal DNA found in rings called plasmids. These plasmids can be extracted from the bacteria and then enzymatically sliced into fragments. After this has been done, DNA taken from other cells or man-made DNA can be attached to these fragments before the plasmid re-forms. The re-formed plasmids, which now carry recombinant DNA, can be taken up by new *E. coli* hosts. In the most successful of these experiments, the foreign genes replicate and function normally within the *E. coli* cells (fig. 5.5).

At the very least, it is hoped that it will be possible to have *E. coli* produce substances needed in large quantities by humans. For example, the gene that codes for human insulin has been placed in *E. coli* and some insulin was produced. Perhaps such bacteria could be grown in huge vats and the insulin could be collected at convenient intervals for packaging and distribution.

Inheritance

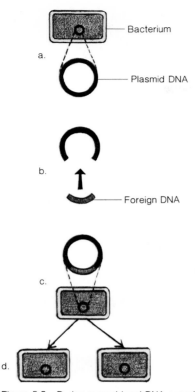

Figure 5.5  During recombinant DNA experimentation
(a) plasmid DNA is removed from *E. coli*; (b) foreign DNA is
incorporated into the plasmid which is (c) then reintroduced
into the bacteria where it (d) functions as a normal gene.
(After Mader, *Inquiry into Life,* 2d edition.)

At most, this technique might offer another means to treat genetic diseases or might even lead to the capability of curing genetic diseases. For example, it might be possible to infect genetically defective individuals with a bacteria or virus that will supply the biological chemical these individuals need. And if genes can eventually be transferred from one human cell to another, then it might be possible to genetically alter a human egg *in vitro* before it is fertilized by a sperm *in vitro*. This possibility will be discussed further in chapter 11.

Some scientists have expressed great concern over DNA recombinant experiments because *E. coli* is a bacterium that normally lives in the human large intestine where it usually causes no harm. Suppose, however, a transformed bacteria carrying recombinant DNA were to escape the laboratory and infect an entire populace. Under these circumstances, it is conceivable that a large number of people could become ill or even die. An *E. coli* that makes insulin might cause nondiabetic individuals to go into insulin shock, for example.

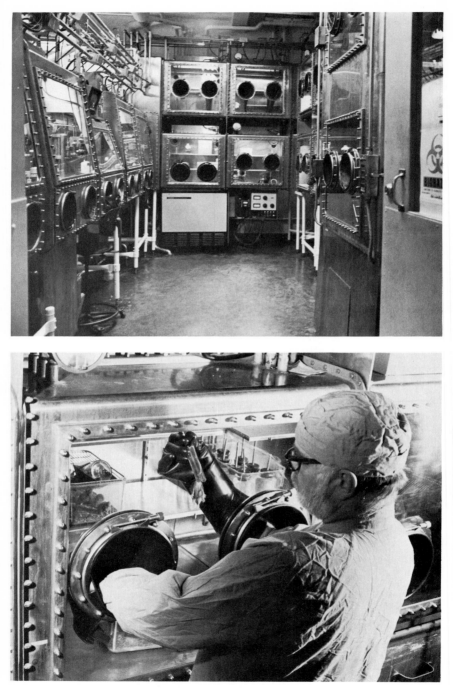

Figure 5.6    P$_4$ laboratory setting. (Source: National Institute of
Allergy and Infectious Diseases, National Institutes of Health.)

Inheritance

For these reasons, scientists have decided that recombinant DNA experiments must be carefully controlled. Scientists, along with officials of the National Institutes of Health, have decided that there are various degrees of danger in plasmid research, depending on the source of the gene involved. If the gene in question is from a lower organism, such as another bacterium, and if the gene is nontoxic to humans, the research is said to be at the $P_1$ level and no restrictions exist. There are ever-increasing safeguards required for $P_2$ - $P_4$ research; $P_4$ research involves the passage of human genes to bacteria capable of infecting humans. For these experiments, the laboratory is supposed to have all possible safeguards that can be devised to prevent infection of personnel. These safeguards cannot be provided in a normal laboratory setting; only special buildings and equipment suffice (fig. 5.6).

The emotional furor over plasmid research seems to be due not only to the fact that this research could be potentially dangerous but also to the fact that we may be entering a new era in which the genotype could possibly be altered and manipulated by science. Cell fusion experiments, such as the man-mouse fusions discussed below, are another type of experiment that will probably contribute to this possibility.

Man-Mouse Cells

Human and mouse cells are mixed together in a laboratory dish and, in the presence of inactivated virus of a special type, they fuse. As the cells grow and divide, some of the human chromosomes are lost and eventually the daughter cells contain only a few human chromosomes (fig. 5.7), each of which can be recognized by their distinctive banding (p. 4). Analysis of the proteins made by the various man-mouse cells can enable scientists to determine which human proteins are to be associated with which human chromosomes. This is a first step toward mapping the human chromosome. A complete map of a chromosome would indicate the order of the genes on the chromosome. Sometimes it is possible to form a man-mouse hybrid in which the human chromosome is shortened, and certain genes are missing. In this way, it is even possible to determine the approximate location of the genes along the chromosome.

It has also been discovered that genes normally inactive in certain types of human cells can be turned on inside a man-mouse hybrid. It is hoped that this phenomenon will enable scientists to determine how genes are controlled within cells. The possibility exists that some genetic diseases are caused by "turned-off" genes rather than defective genes.

Knowing the location of genes on human chromosomes and how they are turned on should increase the likelihood that human genes may be manipulated at will in the future. This possibility is feared by some and looked forward to by others. The social questions involved are in the process of being looked at by all, and both scientists and nonscientists are discussing the propriety of genetic engineering.

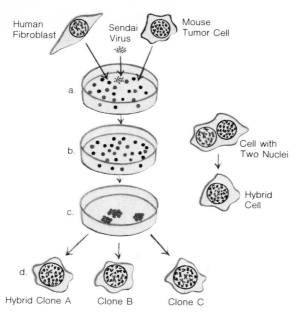

Figure 5.7  (a) In the presence of a Sendai virus, human skin cells sometimes join with mouse tumor cells to give cells with two nuclei (b). (c) Fusion of the nuclei produces hybrid cells that retain all the mouse chromosomes but lose most of the human chromosomes. (d) Each hybrid clone (descendant of a single hybrid cell) has a different complement of human chromosomes which can be studied separately. (After Ruddle, F.S. and Kucherlapati, R.S., "Hybrid Cells and Human Genes," *Scientific American* July 1976.)

## Summary

There is great concern today about environmental mutagens, influences that can bring about mutations in humans. A wide range of mutagens have been detected, including food additives, pesticides, radiation, and industrial chemicals.

Some persons have also expressed concern about modern genetic research particularly recombinant DNA experiments in which portions of a DNA molecule are introduced into host cells, particularly *E. coli* bacteria. Others are hopeful that these experiments will result in *E. coli* cells that can produce chemicals needed by humans. There is also hope that laboratory manipulation of sperm and egg DNA could eventually bring about a cure of human genetic dieseases.

Cell fusion experiments, such as the production of man-mouse hybrids, have furthered the mapping of human chromosomes and increased our knowledge of how genes are internally controlled.

---

## Terms

E. coli
genetic engineering
germinal mutation
in vitro
in vivo
mutagens

mutation
plasmid
radiation
recombinant DNA
somatic mutation

---

## Review

1. What are the two major types of radiation? Which of these is more likely to cause mutations in humans?
2. Name some well-known mutagens.
3. Describe the cellular changes that precede lung cancer in humans.
4. How do in vitro genetic experiments differ from in vivo experiments?
5. Describe two types of in vivo experiments.
6. What is the major concern regarding recombinant DNA experiments?

---

## Further Readings for Part 1

Baer, A. W. 1977. The Genetic Perspective. Philadelphia: W. B. Saunders.

Brown, D. D. 1973. The isolation of genes. Scientific American 229 (9): 20–29.

Grobstein, C. 1977. The recombinant-DNA debate. Scientific American 237 (1): 22.

Lerner, I. M., and Libby, W. 1976. Heredity, Evolution, and Society, 2nd ed. San Francisco: W. H. Freeman & Co.

Mazia, D. 1974. The cell cycle. Scientific American 230 (1): 54.

McKusick, V. A. 1969. Human Genetics, 2nd ed. Englewood Cliffs, N.J.: Prentice-Hall, Inc.

Murray, R. F., et al. 1972. The Genetics, Metabolic and Developmental Aspects of Mental Retardation. Springfield, Ill.: Charles C Thomas, Publishers.

Penrose, L. S. 1973. Outline of Human Genetics. New York: Crane, Russak & Company.

Ruddle, F. H., and Jucherlapati, R. S. 1974. Hybrid cells and human genes. Scientific American 231 (1): 36.

Smith, D. W., and Wilson, A. A. 1973. *The Child with Down's Syndrome*. Philadelphia: W. B. Saunders Co.

Stent, G. S. 1971. *Molecular Genetics: An Introductory Narrative*. San Francisco: W. H. Freeman & Co.

Stern, C. 1973. *Principles of Human Genetics*, 3rd ed. San Francisco: W. H. Freeman & Co.

Sutton, H. E. 1975. *An Introduction to Human Genetics*, 2nd ed. New York: Holt, Rinehart and Winston.

Taylor, J. H. 1958. The duplication of chromosomes. *Scientific American* 198 (6): 36.

Winchester, A. M. 1975. *Human Genetics*. Columbus, Ohio: Charles E. Merrill Publishing Co.

Inheritance

*Part* **2 Human Reproduction**

# Secondary Sex Characteristics

6

The human species is **dimorphic**—its members exist in two different forms. The two forms are male and female, and they are distinguished by the **primary sex characteristics** (the sex organs) and the **secondary sex characteristics** (other physical differences). In everyday life we use the secondary sex characteristics to tell us if we are in the company of a male or female. The secondary sex characteristics develop as a result of hormonal action; the most important of these hormones are the sex hormones produced by the gonads— the ovaries or the testes. The sex chromosomes (XX in females and XY in males) significantly control the development of the sex organs. Recent research suggests that the Y chromosome directs the production of a protein called the **H-Y antigen**[1] and that this protein commands the embryonic nondifferentiated gonads to develop into testes.

Once the embryonic gonads develop into testes, they begin to produce the male sex hormones called androgens. These promote the prenatal development and the maturation of the male organs plus the secondary sex characteristics at puberty.

One theory about sex development in the fetus holds that in the absence of H-Y antigen and subsequent androgen production, the fetus becomes a female. In other words, the embryo, according to this theory, is basically female and/or will automatically develop into a female unless the H-Y antigen and male hormones are present. The sex hormones produced by the ovaries promote the maturation of the female organs plus the secondary sex characteristics at puberty, (fig. 6.1).

Sex hormones act at the cellular level and are believed to enter only those cells that have specific receptors to receive them (fig. 6.2). Once the hormone has combined with the receptor, the complex moves into the nucleus where it binds with a portion of DNA. Thereafter, there is accelerated synthesis of mes-

---

1. The H-Y antigen takes its name from the fact that females produce antibodies against it. To test for maleness, it is possible to suspend a sample of white blood cells in a serum that contains some of these antibodies. If the cells carry H-Y antigen, indicating that the person is a male, the serum antibodies bind with them.

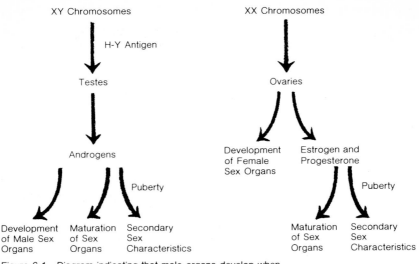

Figure 6.1    Diagram indicating that male organs develop when androgens are present and female organs develop when androgens are absent. Respective sex hormones, however, cause the maturation of sex organs and promote the secondary sex characteristics at puberty.

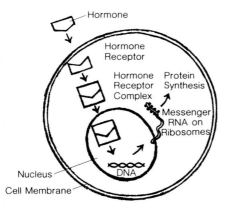

Figure 6.2    Cells that have sex hormone receptors in the cytoplasm are affected by sex hormones. The hormone-receptor complex moves into the nucleus where it activates certain genes leading to transcription and translation. (After Mader, *Inquiry into Life,* 2d edition.)

senger RNA with subsequent protein synthesis. It is believed that each sex hormone promotes the activity of certain genes and it is this action that assists the development of maleness and femaleness.

Sex hormones, like other hormones, reach receptive cells called their target cells by way of the bloodstream. A **hormone** may be defined as a chemical produced by one set of cells but which affects a different set of cells. Hormones are produced by glands called **endocrine glands**, or glands of internal secretion, because their products are distributed in the bloodstream.

## Endocrine Glands

The major endocrine glands of the body are listed in chart 6.1. Figure 6.3 shows their location in the body. The glands of special interest to us are the pituitary gland, the adrenal glands, and the gonads (testes in males and ovaries in females).

**Chart 6.1**

Some Major Endocrine Glands and Their Major Hormones

| Name | Hormone | Function |
| --- | --- | --- |
| *Pituitary gland* | | |
| Anterior | Thyrotropic (TSH) | Stimulates thyroid |
| | Somatotropic (GH) | Stimulates growth |
| | Adrenocorticotropic (ACTH) | Stimulates adrenal cortex |
| | Prolactin (Lactotropic, LTH) | Stimulates milk production |
| | Gonadotropic (FSH) (LH) | Stimulates gonads |
| Posterior | Vasopressin (Antidiuretic, ADH) | Regulates water reabsorption by kidneys |
| | Oxytocin | Milk letdown |
| *Adrenal gland* | | |
| Cortex | Cortisol | Involved in sugar metabolism and relieves stress |
| | Aldosterone | Regulates salt reabsorption by kidneys |
| | Sex hormones | See androgens and estrogen below |
| Medulla | Adrenalin | Fight or flight |
| *Pancreas* | Insulin | Lowers blood sugar |
| *Gonads* | | |
| Testes | Androgens (testosterone) | Promote maturation of sex organs |
| Ovaries | Estrogen and progesterone | Promote and maintain secondary sex characteristics |

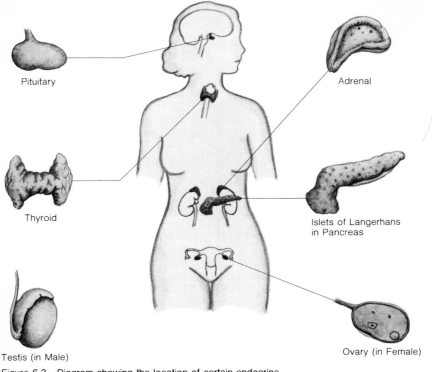

Pituitary

Adrenal

Thyroid

Islets of Langerhans
in Pancreas

Testis (in Male)

Ovary (in Female)

Figure 6.3   Diagram showing the location of certain endocrine
glands in the body. (After Mader, *Inquiry into Life,* 2d edition.)

## Pituitary Gland

The **pituitary gland** is composed of two parts, the **anterior** and **posterior
pituitary**. It lies at the base of the brain and is connected to the **hypothalamus**,
a portion of the brain that has centers for body temperature, sleep, sexual
activity, and emotional states. The hypothalamus controls both the anterior and
posterior pituitary. In fact, it produces two hormones, **vasopressin** and **oxytocin**, which are secreted by the posterior pituitary. These hormones pass from
the hypothalamus to the posterior pituitary by way of nerve fibers (fig. 6.4).
**Oxytocin** is of particular interest to us because it is involved in **lactation**, or
milk production (p. 97), and it stimulates uterine contraction.

The hypothalamus produces **releasing factors** that control the anterior
pituitary. These factors, which pass from the hypothalamus to the anterior pituitary
by way of tiny blood vessels, i.e., capillaries, stimulate the anterior pituitary to
produce and secrete its hormones. Each of the five types of hormones (chart
6.1) made by the anterior pituitary has a name composed of two parts: the first
part indicates a target organ or gland and the last part is the word tropic, which

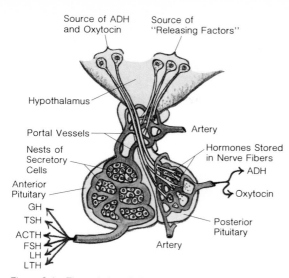

Source of ADH and Oxytocin

Source of "Releasing Factors"

Hypothalamus

Portal Vessels

Artery

Nests of Secretory Cells

Hormones Stored in Nerve Fibers

ADH

Anterior Pituitary

Oxytocin

GH
TSH
ACTH
FSH
LH
LTH

Posterior Pituitary

Artery

Figure 6.4   The anterior pituitary is connected to the hypothalamus by capillaries, while the posterior pituitary is connected by nerves. See chart 6.1 for the full names of the hormones listed here by initials. (After Chaffee and Greisheimer, *Basic Physiology and Anatomy*, 3d ed., 1974. Used by permission of J.B. Lippincott.)

**Chart 6.2**
Master Gland

| Anterior Pituitary Hormone | Gland | Hormone |
|---|---|---|
| ACTH | Adrenal cortex | Cortisol |
| TSH | Thyroid gland | Thyroxin |
| FSH, LH | Gonads | |
| | Testes | Testosterone |
| | Ovaries | Estrogen and progesterone |

means "being drawn to." Since the anterior pituitary produces hormones that regulate other endocrine glands (chart 6.2), it is sometimes called the **master gland** (fig. 6.5).

Adrenal Glands

The **adrenal glands**, located atop the kidneys, have an outer *cortex* and inner *medulla*. Under the influence of *ACTH* the cortex secretes **cortisol**, a very

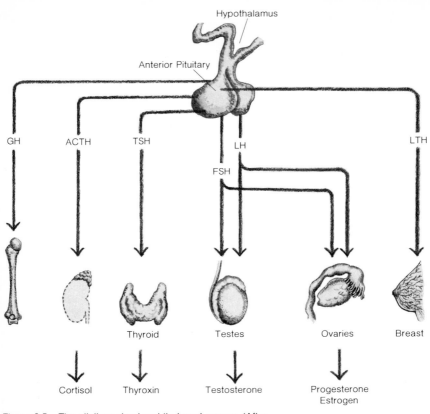

Figure 6.5  The pituitary gland and its target organs. (After
Guillemin, R. and Burgus, R., "The Hormones of the
Hypothalamus," *Scientific American*, Nov. 1972.)

important hormone involved in cellular metabolism. But of more interest to us is the fact that the adrenal cortex also produces a small amount of both male and female sex hormones. Therefore, in males the cortex is a source of female sex hormones and in females it is a source of male hormones. It's possible that estrogen in males and androgen in females have important functions, but it is not known specifically what these functions are. If by chance the adrenal cortex begins to produce a large amount of sex hormones, it can lead to feminization in the male and masculinization in the female.

Gonads

The gonads—testes in the male and ovaries in the female—are controlled by two **gonadotropic hormones**, *FSH* and *LH*, which are produced by the anterior pituitary. These hormones, as we shall see, are named for their action in the female but exist in both sexes, stimulating the appropriate gonads in each. The testes produce the male sex hormones called **androgens**, of which the most potent is **testosterone**. The ovaries produce the female sex hormones called **estrogen** and **progesterone**. The level of sex hormones in the body or, for that matter, the level of most hormones, is regulated by a mechanism called feedback control.

## Feedback Control

By means of feedback control a system can regulate itself provided that it has a sensing device. Consider a home furnace and thermostat by which the temperature of individual rooms can be maintained using feedback control. The furnace produces heat and when the temperature of a room reaches the temperature indicated on the thermostat, the sensing device in this case, the furnace is automatically shut off. On the other hand, when the temperature falls below that indicated on the thermostat, the furnace produces heat again (fig. 6.6). The production of heat by a furnace must be regulated because it is not known in advance how the outside temperature will affect how much heat will be needed to maintain the desired temperature of the room.

Similarly, the need for hormones may fluctuate depending on the body's need. When the level of a hormone is sufficient, the gland producing the hormone is shut off; when the level of the hormone is insufficient, the gland begins to produce it again.

Sex hormone levels are maintained by a feedback control (fig. 6.7) system that involves the hypothalamus, the anterior pituitary, and the gonads. The hypothalamic releasing factors stimulate the anterior pituitary to produce the gonadotropic hormones that travel to the gonads by way of the circulatory system. In the male, the testes produce testosterone and in the female the ovaries produce estrogen and progesterone. These hormones promote the

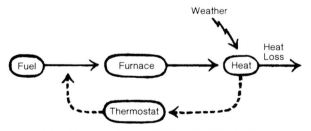

Figure 6.6   A furnace produces heat and when the heat reaches a certain level, the thermostat (a sensing device) turns off the furnace. When heat is needed, the thermostat turns on the furnace. Since the product (heat) is controlling its own production, this is termed feedback control.

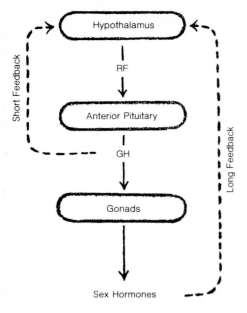

RF = Releasing Factors
GH = Gonadotrophic Hormones

Figure 6.7   The level of sex hormones in the body controls the production of hypothalamic releasing factors and thus sex hormonal levels are regulated by feedback control.

development of the primary and secondary sex characteristics, but they also exert feedback control over the hypothalamus and anterior pituitary. When the sex hormones reach a certain level in the body, the hypothalamus stops producing releasing factors and the pituitary stops producing gonadotropic hormones. When the level of sex hormones falls, then, the hypothalamus again produces releasing factors, reactivating the system.

As indicated by figure 6.8, the hypothalamus can also be controlled by the level of gonadotropic hormones in the body. In other words, both the level of sex hormones and the level of gonadotropic hormones serve to stimulate or depress the production of releasing factors by the hypothalamus as appropriate.

## Secondary Sex Characteristics

During the teenage years, at the time of **puberty**, the sex organs mature and the secondary sex characteristics begin to appear. The cause of puberty is related to the level of sex hormones in the body. It is now recognized that the *hypothalamic-pituitary-gonad* system functions long before puberty, but the level of hormones is low (fig. 6.8) because the hypothalamus is supersensitive to

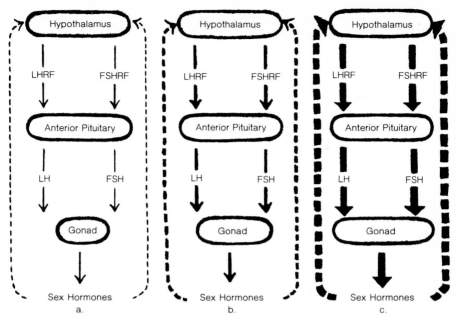

Figure 6.8 (a) Before puberty the level of sex hormones is low because the hypothalamus is very sensitive to feedback control. (b) At puberty the sensitivity of the hypothalamus decreases and therefore the level of sex hormones increases in the body. Decreased sensitivity continues until (c) the adult level of sex hormones is reached.

feedback control. At the start of puberty, the hypothalamus becomes less sensitive to feedback control and begins to increase its production of releasing factors, causing the pituitary and the gonads to increase their production of hormones. The sensitivity of the hypothalamus continues to decrease until the gonadotropic and sex hormones reach the adult level.

The sex hormones, in conjunction with other hormones, have a profound effect on the body during puberty (fig. 6.9). There is an acceleration of growth leading to changes in height, weight, fat distribution, and body proportions. Males commonly experience a growth spurt later than females; thus, they grow for a longer period of time (fig. 6.10). This means that males are generally taller than females and have broader shoulders and longer legs relative to trunk length. Androgens are responsible for the greater muscular development in males and estrogens are responsible for a greater accumulation of fat beneath the skin in females. The latter causes females to have a more rounded appearance than males. In general, it can be assumed that the sex hormones are responsible for these and the other secondary sex characteristics.

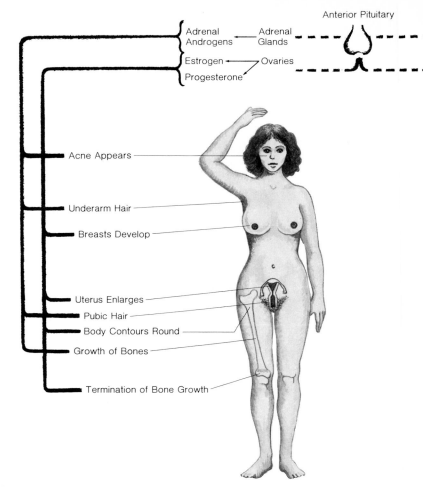

Figure 6.9   Diagram illustrating the many effects of both male
and female sex hormones in both sexes. The adrenal cortex is
a source of androgens in females and of estrogens in males.
(Source: Redrawn after a CIBA Pharmaceutical Company
illustration by Dr. Frank H. Vetter.)

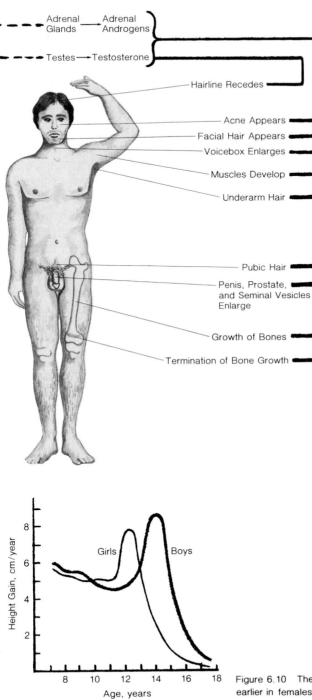

Adrenal Glands → Adrenal Androgens

Testes → Testosterone

Hairline Recedes

Acne Appears

Facial Hair Appears

Voicebox Enlarges

Muscles Develop

Underarm Hair

Pubic Hair

Penis, Prostate, and Seminal Vesicles Enlarge

Growth of Bones

Termination of Bone Growth

Girls   Boys

Figure 6.10   The growth spurt tends to occur earlier in females than in males.

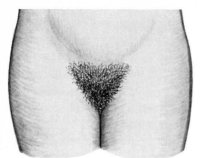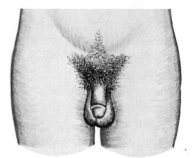

Figure 6.11  In females, the upper border of pubic hair is usually horizontal, while in males pubic hair tapers toward the navel.

### Distribution of Hair

Both males and females develop **axillary** (underarm) and **pubic**[2] hair. In females the upper border of pubic hair is horizontal and in males it tapers toward the navel (fig. 6.11). Males develop noticeable hair on the face, chest, and even occasionally on other regions of the body such as the back, whereas females do not. Oil- and sweat-producing glands become active in both sexes, and **acne** may accompany puberty due to clogged oil-producing glands.

### Voice

The deeper voice of males is due to the fact that they have a larger larynx (voice box) with longer vocal cords. Since the Adam's apple is a part of the voice box, it is usually more prominent in males than in females.

### Breasts

Early growth of the breasts, or mammary glands, is referred to as ''budding'' of the breasts. Budding is followed by development of **lobes**, the functional portions of the breast, and deposition of adipose (fat) tissue that gives breasts their adult shape.

A breast contains 15 to 25 lobes, each with its own **milk duct** that opens at the **nipple**. The nipple is surrounded by a pigmented area called the **areola**. Hair and sweat glands are absent from the nipples and areola, but glands are present that secrete a saliva-resisting lubricant to protect the nipples, particularly during nursing. Smooth muscle fibers in the region of the areola may cause the nipple to become erect in response to stimulation.

Within each lobe, the milk duct divides into numerous **alveolar ducts** that can end in blind sacs called **alveoli** (fig. 6.12). The alveoli are made up of the cells that can produce milk.

2. Pubic or pubis refers to the front of the pelvic girdle (p. 98).

Human Reproduction

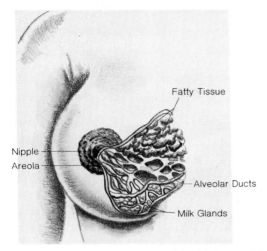

Figure 6.12    The female breast contains lobules consisting of ducts and alveoli. The alveoli, lined by milk-producing cells, are more numerous in the lactating breast.

Estrogen and progesterone are required for lobe development. It is believed that estrogen causes proliferation of ducts and that both estrogen and progesterone bring about alveolar development. The abundance of these hormones during pregnancy means that the alveoli proliferate at this time. There are ducts but few alveoli in the nonlactating breast and there are many ducts and alveoli in the lactating breast.

There is no production of milk during pregnancy. The hormone **prolactin** (lactotropic hormone) is needed for lactation to begin, and the production of this hormone is suppressed because of the feedback control that the increased amount of estrogen and progesterone during pregnancy has on the pituitary (p. 152). Once the baby is delivered, however, the pituitary does begin secreting prolactin. It takes a couple of days for milk production to begin and, in the meantime, the breasts produce a watery, yellowish-white fluid called **colostrum**, which has the same composition as milk except that it contains more protein and less fat.

The continued production of milk requires a suckling child. When a breast is *suckled,* the nerve endings in the areola are stimulated and a nerve impulse travels from the nipples to the hypothalamus, which directs the pituitary gland to release the hormone oxytocin. When this hormone arrives at the breasts, it causes contraction of the lobules so that milk flows into the ducts (called milk letdown), where it may be drawn out of the nipple by the suckling child. The more suckling, the more oxytocin released and the more milk there is for the child (fig. 6.13).

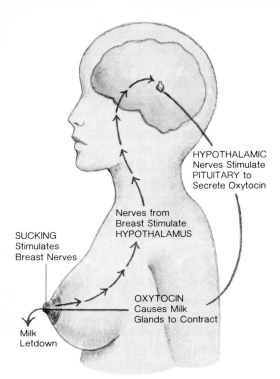

HYPOTHALAMIC
Nerves Stimulate
PITUITARY to
Secrete Oxytocin

Nerves from
Breast Stimulate
HYPOTHALAMUS

SUCKING
Stimulates
Breast Nerves

OXYTOCIN
Causes Milk
Glands to Contract

Milk
Letdown

Figure 6.13   Suckling reflex. Suckling stimulates release of
oxytocin from the pituitary and milk letdown.

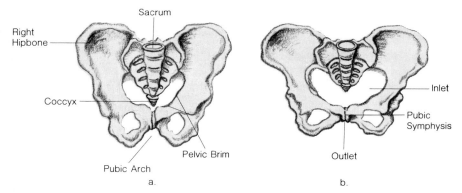

Sacrum

Right
Hipbone

Coccyx

Pelvic Brim

Pubic Arch

a.

Inlet

Pubic
Symphysis

Outlet

b.

Figure 6.14   Human pelvic girdle in (a) male and (b) female.

## Pelvis

The pelvis is a bony cavity formed by the hip bones and the sacrum and coccyx at the back (fig. 6.14). In females, a pelvic cavity outlet that can accommodate the passage of a baby's head allows a natural birth. During puberty, the pelvic girdle enlarges in females so that the pelvic cavity usually has a larger relative size compared to males. This means that females have wider hips than males and that the thighs converge at a greater angle toward the knees. Because the female pelvis tilts forward, females tend to have protruding buttocks, a more pronounced lower back curve, and an abdominal bulge.

---

**Summary**

The secondary sex characteristics are controlled by hormones, notably the sex hormones produced by the gonads. Sex hormones, which act at the cellular level, are believed to turn on certain genes. Production is controlled by a feedback system involving the hypothalamus and anterior pituitary.

Increasing desensitivity at puberty causes the hypothalamus to increase its production of releasing factors, which causes the anterior pituitary to increase its production of gonadotropic hormones. The gonadotropic hormones stimulate the gonads to produce the sex hormones with the subsequent development of the secondary sex characteristics involving distribution of hair, voice depth, breast development, and pelvic size.

---

**Terms**

| | |
|---|---|
| adrenal glands | oxytocin |
| androgens | pelvis |
| dimorphism | pituitary gland |
| endocrine glands | primary sex characteristics |
| estrogen | progesterone |
| feedback control | prolactin (lactotropic hormone) |
| gonadotropic hormones | puberty |
| hormone | releasing factors |
| H-Y antigen | secondary sex characteristics |
| hypothalamus | testosterone |
| mammary gland | |

**Review**

1. Describe a theory that explains why a male baby develops instead of a female baby.
2. Explain how sex hormones work at the cellular level.
3. Define a hormone and name the major endocrine glands and their hormones.
4. Describe the anatomical relationship of the pituitary gland to the hypothalamus and describe how the hypothalamus ''controls'' the pituitary gland.
5. Name the six hormones produced by the anterior pituitary and explain why the anterior pituitary is called the master gland.
6. Describe the principle of feedback control.
7. How does feedback control operate in relation to the hypothalamic-pituitary-gonad system?
8. What are the secondary sex characteristics in males and females? When do they develop? What factors cause them to develop?
9. Describe the anatomy of the breast. Name the hormones needed for breast development and milk production and release.

# Male Reproductive Anatomy

**7**

In advanced forms of sexual reproduction, two gametes, the sperm and the egg, contribute chromosomes to the new individual. The sperm are small and swims to the egg, a much larger cell containing food for the developing embryo. It seems reasonable that there should be a large number of sperm to ensure that a few will find an egg. Correspondingly in humans, the male continually produces a large number of sperm that are temporarily stored before being released.

The primary sex organs of the male (fig. 7.1 and chart 7.1) may be categorized as follows:

**Essential organs**: Testis (pl. testes) produces sperm and secretes androgens, particularly testosterone.

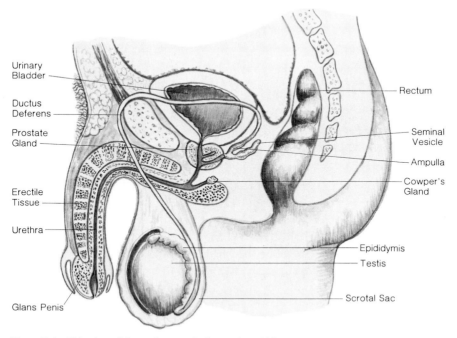

Figure 7.1   Side view of the male reproductive system. (After Mader, *Inquiry into Life,* 2d edition.)

**Chart 7.1**
Male Reproductive System

| Organ | Function |
| --- | --- |
| Testes | Produce sperm and sex hormones |
| Epididymides | Maturation and some storage of sperm |
| Ductus deferentia | Conduct and store sperm |
| Seminal vesicles | Contributes to seminal fluid |
| Prostate gland | Contributes to seminal fluid |
| Urethra | Conducts sperm |
| Cowper's glands | Contribute to seminal fluid |
| Penis | Organ of copulation |

**Excretory ducts:** The epididymis (pl. epididymides), ductus or vas deferens (pl. ductus deferentia), ejaculatory ducts, and urethra store and/or transport sperm (spermatozoa). Penis is copulatory organ.

**Accessory glands**: Seminal vesicles, prostate gland, and Cowper's glands contribute secretions to seminal fluid.

## Testes

The **testes** are paired oval-shaped organs measuring about two inches in length and one inch in diameter. They begin their development inside the abdominal cavity, but under the influence of testosterone they descend into the **scrotal sacs**, which lie outside the body. If by chance the testes do not descend and the male is not treated by administration of testosterone or operated on to place the testes in the **scrotum**, sterility follows. The reason for this type of **sterility**, the inability to produce offspring, is that normal sperm production does not occur at body temperature; a cooler temperature is required. Assuming that a male is wearing loose clothing, the scrotal sacs will hold the testes close to the groin or away from the groin as appropriate to maintain a temperature of about 95°. The sacs can do this because they have layers of muscle that automatically adjust their degree of contraction in response to surrounding temperatures without the man's conscious control. Tight clothing that squeezes the scrotum against the body can deter normal sperm production.

A longitudinal cut (fig. 7.2) shows that internally each testis is composed of compartments called **lobules**. Each lobule contains 1–3 tightly coiled **seminiferous tubules** separated by **interstitial cells**. Altogether, these tubules have a combined length of approximately 750 feet. A microscopic cross section (fig. 7.2b) through a tubule shows that it is packed with cells undergoing spermatogenesis. These cells are derived from undifferentiated germ cells, called **spermatogonia**, that lie just inside the outer membrane and divide mitotically

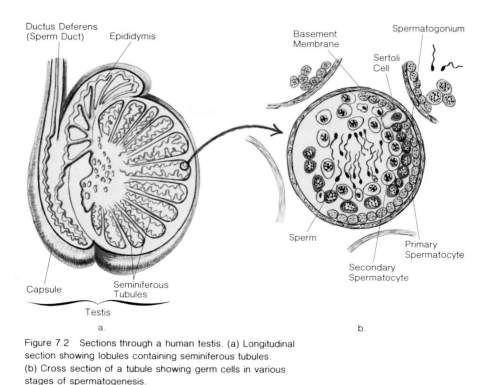

Figure 7.2   Sections through a human testis. (a) Longitudinal section showing lobules containing seminiferous tubules. (b) Cross section of a tubule showing germ cells in various stages of spermatogenesis.

always producing new spermatogonia. **Germ cell** is a generalized term for those cells in males and females that give rise to the sex cells. Some spermatogonia move away from the outer membrane and increase in size and become **primary spermatocytes** that undergo meiosis, a process described on page 9. Primary spermatocytes have 46 chromosomes and divide into **secondary spermatocytes** that each have 23 chromosomes. Secondary spermatocytes divide to give **spermatids** that also have 23 chromosomes, but these are single chromosomes. Spermatids are transformed into **spermatozoa**, or mature sperm cells.

Notice in fig. 7.2b that developing germ cells lie progressively further away from the outer membrane as they mature. Spermatogonia are near the membrane, followed by spermatocytes and spermatids. Sperm are in the center of the tubule with their tails projecting into the lumen, or internal cavity. Throughout the entire process of spermatogenesis, the germ cells are in intimate contact with **sertoli cells** that extend from the membrane to the lumen, apparently assisting and nourishing the germ cells as they mature. Portions of the same tubule are at different stages of spermatogenesis, a process that takes 16 days to complete.

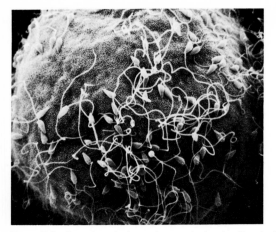

Figure 7.3 Scanning electron micrograph showing the single egg surrounded by the numerous and smaller sperm. (Source: "Sea Urchin Sperm-Egg Interactions Studied with the Scanning Electron Microscope," Tegner, M.J., and Epel, D., *Science*, vol. 179, pp. 685–88, fig. 2, Feb. 1973.)

Spermatozoa (fig. 1.13) have three distinct parts: a head, a mid-piece, and a tail. The *tail* contains contractile filaments that propel the sperm at a rate of up to 1 inch per second and the *mid-piece* contains energy-producing organelles. The *head* contains the 23 chromosomes within a nucleus. The tip of the nucleus is covered by a cap called the **acrosome** that is believed to contain enzymes needed for fertilization to take place. The human egg is surrounded by several layers of cells and a membrane called the **zona pellucida**. The acrosome enzymes are believed to play a role in allowing the sperm to reach the surface of the egg so that one can enter. Each acrosome probably contains so little enzyme that it requires the action of many sperm to allow just one to actually enter the egg. This may explain why so many sperm (fig. 7.3) are required for the process of fertilization. The normal human male may produce several hundred million sperm per day, assuring an adequate number for fertilization to take place.

Interstitial Cells

Androgens are believed to be produced by cells, called *interstitial cells*, that lie between the seminiferous tubules (fig. 7.2b). Androgens, especially testosterone, promote the maturation of the primary sex characteristics (p. 85) and the development and maintenance of the secondary sex characteristics (p. 92) in males. Androgen production is under the direct control of the anterior pituitary gonadotropic hormone LH. Since LH is named for its action in females, it is sometimes given the name **Interstitial Cell Stimulating Hormone** (ICSH) in the male. Evidence suggests that the interstitial cells also produce estrogen either directly or as a by-product of testosterone production. Some investigators believe that estrogen has an important function in the feedback control of sex hormone levels in the male, discussed following.

## Hormonal Regulation in the Male

While LH promotes the production of androgens by the interstitial cells, the other gonadotropic hormone, FSH, promotes spermatogenesis in the seminiferous tubules. The hypothalamus (p.88) has ultimate control of the testes' sexual functions, however, because the hypothalamus secretes releasing factors that stimulate the anterior pituitary to produce the gonadotropic hormones (fig. 7.4).

All of the hormones mentioned are involved in a feedback process that maintains the production of sperm and androgens at a fairly constant level. The hypothalamus produces releasing factors that travel to the anterior pituitary by way of small blood vessels called capillaries. The releasing factors cause the anterior pituitary to produce ICSH and FSH. ICSH and FSH travel in the bloodstream to the testes where ICSH stimulates the interstitial cells to produce androgens and where FSH stimulates the tubules to produce sperm. When the amount of testosterone in the blood reaches a certain level, it causes the

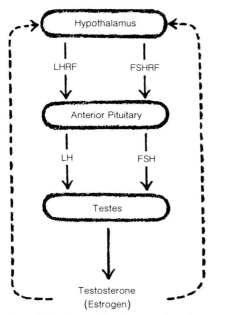

Figure 7.4   Diagram illustrating the hypothalamic-pituitary-gonad system as it functions in the male.

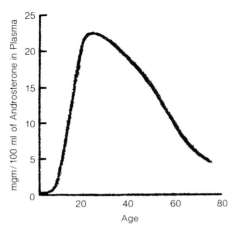

Figure 7.5   Level of testosterone in males according to age.

hypothalamus to decrease the secretion of releasing factor and the anterior pituitary to decrease its secretion of ICSH. Consequently, the interstitial cells temporarily slow down testosterone production. Then, as the level of testosterone in the blood falls, the hypothalamus increases its secretion of ICSH releasing factor and the entire process begins again. It should be emphasized that there are no great fluctuations of testosterone level in the male and the feedback process in this case acts to maintain testosterone at a normal level.

We have explained a feedback process in regard to testosterone but not in regard to sperm production. Presumably, the secretion of FSH releasing factor and FSH is also controlled by a feedback mechanism. Some investigators have suggested that estrogen, produced by the testes, is the inhibiting hormone for this feedback cycle. As mentioned previously, the exact function of estrogen in males is unclear at this time.

In general, a younger man produces more testosterone than an older man (fig. 7.5). Men may begin to exhibit decreasing sexual functions in their late forties and fifties. This decrease is called the **male climacteric** and may at times be accompanied by hot flashes, feelings of suffocation, and psychic disorders similar to those experienced by women during the menopause (p. 122).[1]

## Excretory Ducts
Sperm are made in the testes, but they mature in the **epididymides** (fig. 7.1), which are tightly coiled tubules about 20 feet in length that lie just outside the testes. Maturation seems to be required in order for the sperm to be capable of swimming and thus able to fertilize the egg. Also, it is possible that defective

1. A. C. Guyton, *Textbook of Medical Physiology* (Philadelphia: W. B. Saunders, 1976), p. 1083.

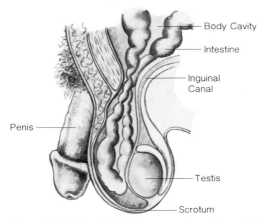

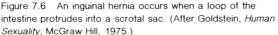

Figure 7.6 An inguinal hernia occurs when a loop of the intestine protrudes into a scrotal sac. (After Goldstein, *Human Sexuality*, McGraw Hill, 1975.)

sperm are removed during the 2–4 days that the sperm normally reside in the epididymides. Each epididymis joins with a **ductus** (vas) **deferens**, which ascends through a canal called the **inguinal canal** and enters the abdomen where it curves around the bladder to open into a short ejaculatory duct. The two **ejaculatory ducts** empty into the urethra. Sperm are stored in the ductus deferentia, which have expanded portions called **ampullae**. They pass from the ductus deferentia into the ejaculatory ducts and **urethra** only during ejaculation, which we will discuss below.

Spermatic Cords

The testes are suspended in the scrotum by the **spermatic cords**, each of which consists of connective tissue and muscle fibers enclosing the ductus deferens, blood vessels, and nerves. The region of the inguinal canal, where the spermatic cord passes into the abdomen, remains a weak point in the abdominal wall. As such, it is frequently the site of a **hernia**. A hernia is an opening or separation of some part of the abdominal wall through which a portion of internal organs, usually the intestine, is apt to protrude (fig. 7.6).

Urogenital System

The urinary system and the reproductive system are sometimes discussed simultaneously under the heading **urogenital system**. This is most appropriate in males because the urethra serves as the passageway for both urine and semen (p. 109). In the *urinary system* (fig. 7.7), urine, made by the kidneys, goes to the bladder by way of the **ureters**. After storage in the bladder, urine passes to the outside by way of the urethra. In the reproductive system, sperm, made

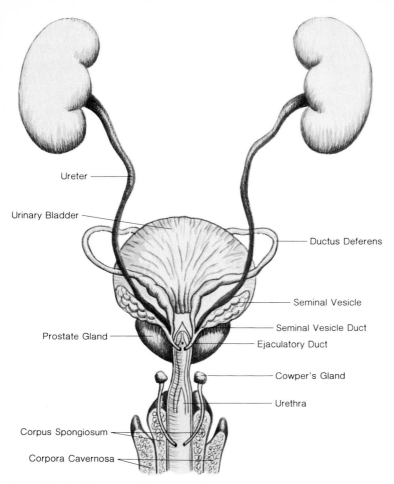

Figure 7.7   Posterior view of the urogenital system in males.

in the testes, mature in the epididiymides before *storage* in the ductus deferentia. When the sperm leave the ductus deferentia they *pass* by way of the ejaculatory ducts into the urethra before being expelled. As this is occurring, the passageway between the bladder and the urethra is closed off by a circulatory muscle called a sphincter.

## Accessory Glands

At the time of ejaculation (p. 111), sperm leave the penis in a fluid called **seminal fluid**. This fluid is produced by three types of glands—the seminal vesicles, the prostate gland, and Cowper's glands. The **seminal vesicles** lie at the base of the bladder and have ducts that empty into the ejaculatory ducts. The **prostate gland** is a single, doughnut-shaped gland that surrounds the upper portion of the urethra just below the bladder. In older men, the prostate may enlarge and cut off the urethra, making urination painful and difficult. This condition may be treated medically and surgically. **Cowper's glands** are pea-sized organs that lie posterior to the prostate on either side of the urethra.

When sperm pass from the ductus deferentia, the accessory glands provide them with a fluid that has various components; each component of seminal fluid seems to have a particular function. Sperm are more viable in a basic solution and seminal fluid, which is white and milky in appearance, has a basic pH. Swimming sperm require energy and seminal fluid contains the sugar fructose that presumably serves as an energy source. There is even a coagulator that clots the **semen** (sperm + seminal fluid), possibly to help prevent leakage of sperm from the vagina, and a decoagulator that unclots the semen again. Seminal fluid also contains prostaglandins, chemicals that cause the uterus to contract. Some scientists now believe that uterine contraction is necessary to propel the sperm and that the sperm only swim when they are in the vicinity of the egg.

Fertility

There may be as many as 400 million or more sperm expelled during ejaculation. This represents 120 million sperm per each ml (millimeter) of ejaculate since the ejaculate is normally about 3.5 ml of semen. When the number of sperm in each ml falls below 10 to 20 million, the male is likely to be infertile. The reason why so many sperm might be required for fertilization has already been discussed on page 104.

Though sperm can live for many weeks in the male genital ducts, once they are ejaculated in the semen their maximal life span is about 24 to 72 hours at body temperature. Semen can be stored longer at a lower temperature and, if frozen, can be preserved for years. Most major cities now have sperm banks in which it is possible to store semen for later use.

Although seminal fluid has many functions, it is not required for the process of fertilization. However, exposure to fluids within the female tract for at least one to two hours does seem to be required before fertilization can take place. Ability of sperm to fertilize is called **capacitation** and it seems to depend on some unknown substances in the vagina and uterus that stimulate final maturation of the sperm so that fertilization can take place.

## Penis

The **penis** has a long shaft and enlarged tip called the **glans penis**. In uncircumcised males (fig. 7.8), the glans penis is covered by a loose-fitting hood of skin. In circumcised males (fig. 7.8b), this hood—called the **foreskin**—has been surgically removed. Jews and Moslems routinely circumcise male infants for

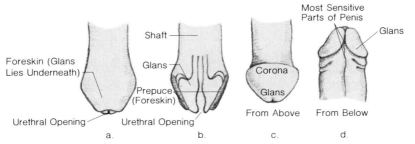

Figure 7.8 (a) Uncircumcised penis. (b) Longitudinal section through an uncircumcised penis. (c) Circumcised penis from above and (d) from below.

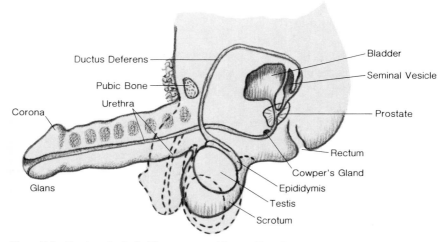

Figure 7.9 Erect penis. Dotted lines represent the position of the flaccid penis and relaxed scrotum.

religious reasons. There are also medical reasons for circumcision. Glands under the foreskin discharge a white, cheesy substance called **smegma**. If smegma accumulates under the foreskin, irritation and infection can result. It has also been suggested, but not proven, that there is less penile cancer in circumcised males and less cervical cancer in their mates. Even so, there are those who do not favor circumcision on the ground that the foreskin may have an important function that has yet to be realized and that unnecessary surgery should not be done in any case. There is also the possibility that sexual performance could possibly be affected by circumcision in some individuals.

The penis is the copulatory organ of males. During sexual arousal, the penis becomes erect (fig. 7.9) and capable of being placed into the vagina of a female. **Erection**, which is discussed in detail on page 142, is dependent on an increased flow of blood to and a decreased flow of blood away from the penis. The penis contains **erectile tissue** that expands when filled with blood; this accounts for the fact that the penis becomes wider, longer, and firmer during an erection. In its flaccid state, the penis averages 3 to 4 inches in length and 1 inch in diameter. In an erect state, it averages 6 to 7 inches in length and 1½ inches in diameter. The size of the flaccid penis is actually unimportant because a small penis enlarges to a greater extent than a large penis. Also, the muscles at the base of the vagina can be constricted (p. 146) to adjust its size to that of the penis. In any case, a female receives stimulation through friction of the penis against the walls of the exterior opening of the vagina.

If sexual arousal reaches a certain level, ejaculation follows an erection. During **ejaculation** semen, which contains sperm and seminal fluid, spurts from the tip of the penis at the opening of the urethra. The force of ejaculation varies and is dependent on the particular sexual circumstances and on the particular anatomy of the male. Prior to ejaculation, a mucus secretion from the Cowper's glands may leak from the penis and this may contain numerous sperm.

An erection lasts for only a limited amount of time. Upon detumescence, which follows ejaculation and/or the loss of sexual arousal, the penis returns to its normal flaccid state. Following ejaculation, a male may typically experience a period of time, called the refractory period, during which stimulation does not bring about an erection.

---

## Summary

The gonads of a male are the testes located in the scrotal sacs. Inside the testes, spermatogenesis occurs within seminiferous tubules, which are separated by interstitial cells where the male sex hormones, the androgens, are produced. Under the control of FSH produced by the anterior pituitary, spermatogenesis, which involves meiosis, occurs continuously. Consequently, the male produces a very large number of sperm each having 23 chromosomes. Androgen production is under the control of ICSH, another gonadotropic hormone. Feedback control in the male results in little fluctuation of testosterone or sperm production.

Sperm mature in the epididymides and are stored in the ductus deferentia. At the time of sexual excitement, they move from ductus deferentia to the urethra located within the penis. Several glands (seminal vesicles, prostate gland, and Cowper's glands) contribute to seminal fluid, which is the medium for sperm that pass from the penis during ejaculation. Four hundred million or more sperm may be found in semen.

The penis contains erectile tissue that fills with blood, enabling the penis to become erect so that sexual intercourse might take place.

## Terms

capacitation

circumcision

Cowper's glands

detumescence

ductus deferentia (ductus deferens)

ejaculation

epididymides (epididymis)

erection

interstitial cells

penis

prostate gland

scrotum

semen

seminal fluid

seminal vesicles

seminiferous tubules

testes

urethra

## Review

1. Name two functions of the testes and the part of the organ associated with each function.
2. Explain the hypothalamic-pituitary-gonad relationship in males.
3. Name the glands that produce seminal fluid. Are these glands endocrine glands?
4. State the path of sperm prior to and during ejaculation.
5. Give the normal sperm count per ejaculation. Offer reasons why the sperm count is so high.
6. What organ in males serves to transport both urine and semen?

Human Reproduction

# Female Reproductive Anatomy

# 8

In humans, the female typically produces only one egg a month and this one egg awaits the swimming sperm. Should fertilization occur, the developing zygote implants itself in a specially prepared organ where development proceeds until birth occurs.

The primary sex organs of the female (chart 8.1 and fig. 8.1) may be categorized as follows:

**Essential organs**: Ovaries that produce eggs and the sex hormones, estrogen and progesterone.

**Accessory organs**: Oviducts (uterine or Fallopian tubes) where fertilization occurs; uterus, where development occurs; and vagina, the organ of copulation.

**External genitals**: Mons pubis, clitoris, labia majora, and labia minora.

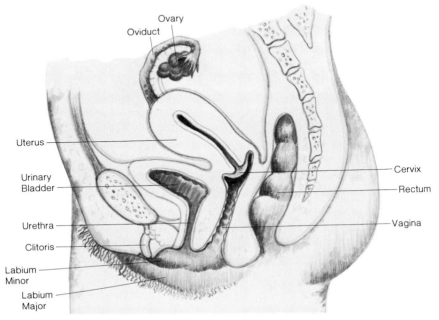

Figure 8.1   Side view of female reproductive organs. (After Mader, *Inquiry into Life,* 2d edition.)

**Chart 8.1**
Female Reproduction System

| Organ | Function |
| --- | --- |
| Ovaries | Produce egg and sex hormones |
| Oviducts (Fallopian tubes) | Conduct egg |
| Uterus (womb) | Location of developing baby |
| Vagina | Copulatory organ |
| Clitoris | Sexual response |

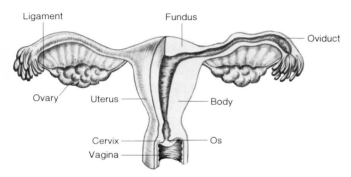

Figure 8.2   Front view of female reproductive organs. (After Mader, *Inquiry into Life,* 2d edition.)

## Ovaries

There are two **ovaries**, one on each side of the upper pelvic cavity. Each ovary ranges in size from 1 to 1½ inches in length and is attached to the uterus and pelvic wall by ligaments (fig. 8.2).

A longitudinal section through an ovary (fig. 8.3) shows that it is made up of an outer **cortex** and inner **medulla**. The cortex contains ovarian **follicles** at various stages of maturation. A female is born with a large number of immature follicles (400,000 in both ovaries), each containing a germ cell surrounded by a layer of nongerminal cells. Only a small number of these follicles (about 400) will ever mature because a female produces only one egg per month during her reproductive years. Since follicles are present at birth, they age as the woman ages. This has been given as a reason why an older woman is more apt to produce a child with a genetic defect.

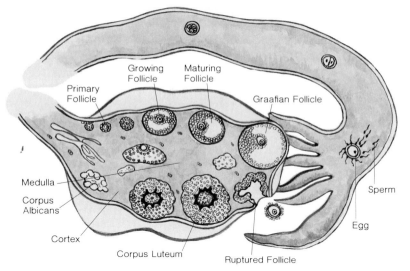

Figure 8.3   Longitudinal section of ovary showing the
development and maturation of a follicle; ovulation; formation,
and degeneration of corpus luteum.

## Oogenesis

During the reproductive years, one follicle a month undergoes complete maturation, developing from a **primary** to a **secondary** to a **Graafian follicle**.
Meiosis (fig. 1.14) in the female begins with a primary oocyte that divides meiot-
ically into two daughter cells, each having 23 chromosomes. However, one of
these cells, called the **secondary oocyte**, receives almost all the cytoplasm,
nutrients, and enzymes. The other cell is a **polar body** that disintegrates or
divides to give two polar bodies that die. If fertilization takes place, the secondary
oocyte divides to give a nucleus that combines with the sperm nucleus and
another polar body that disintegrates.

Within the ovary, a **primary follicle** contains a primary oocyte surrounded
by a large number of follicular cells. A **secondary follicle** contains the secondary oocyte pushed to one side of a fluid-filled cavity. In the **Graafian follicle**,
the fluid-filled cavity increases to the point that the follicle wall balloons out on
the surface of the ovary and bursts, releasing the secondary oocyte surrounded
by a thick membrane, the zona pellucida, and a few cells. This is referred to
as ovulation and for the sake of convenience the released germ cell is called
an **ovum**, or egg. Actually, the second meiotic division does not take place
unless fertilization occurs.

Prior to ovulation, the follicle produces estrogen (and some progesterone). Following ovulation, the follicle is converted into the yellowish **corpus luteum**, which produces progesterone (and some estrogen). If fertilization does not take place, the corpus luteum degenerates into the **corpus albicans**, a whitish scar. If fertilization does take place, the corpus luteum persists for about six months before degenerating.

*Ovarian cycle.* The monthly maturation of a follicle is called the **ovarian cycle**, and this cycle is under the control of the anterior pituitary hormones, **Follicular Stimulating Hormone** (*FSH*) and **Luteinizing Hormone** (*LH*). It is clear from the names of these hormones that FSH may be associated with the maturation of a follicle and that LH may be associated with the functioning of the corpus luteum; from this it might be suspected that the ovarian cycle has two parts, as discussed following.

## Hormonal Regulation in the Female

The gonadotropic and sex hormones are not present in constant amounts in the female and instead are secreted at different rates (fig. 8.4) during a monthly ovarian cycle that usually lasts 28 days but may vary widely. For simplicity's sake, it is most convenient to assume that during the first half of a 28-day cycle the hypothalamus is primarily secreting **FSH releasing factor**, the anterior pituitary is secreting FSH, and the follicle in the ovary is secreting estrogen. Just as FSH releasing factor has caused the anterior pituitary to begin producing FSH, so FSH has brought about follicle development in the ovary. As the blood estrogen level rises, it exerts feedback control (fig. 8.5) over the hypothalamus and anterior pituitary so that this **follicular phase** comes to an end. A sudden surge of LH production causes ovulation to occur on the fourteenth day of a 28-day cycle.[1] During the last half of the ovarian cycle, the hypothalamus is producing **LH releasing factor**, the anterior pituitary is producing LH, and the corpus luteum is secreting progesterone. The LH releasing factor has caused the anterior pituitary to produce LH, which in turn promoted conversion of the follicle into the corpus luteum. As the blood progesterone level rises, it exerts feedback control over the hypothalamus and the anterior pituitary so that this **luteal phase** comes to an end. Then, the corpus luteum degenerates.

1. Ovulation occurs on the fourteenth day prior to the first day of menstruation. Only in a twenty-eight day cycle would this be the fourteenth day counting from day one.

Human Reproduction

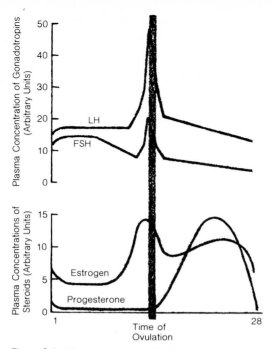

Figure 8.4 Hormone concentration levels accompanying the ovarian cycle.

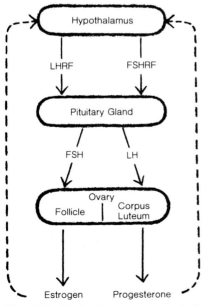

Figure 8.5 The level of sex hormones in the female is under the control of feedback regulation.

The female sex hormones, estrogen and progesterone, have numerous functions (chart 8.2). Some of these functions have been discussed in chapter 6, but one important function still to be discussed is the effect that these hormones have on the uterus. Since the uterus has been classified as an accessory organ, description of the accessory organs follows.

---

**Chart 8.2**
Effects of Female Sex Steroids*

---

Effects of estrogens

---

1. Growth of ovaries and follicles
2. Growth and maintenance of the smooth muscle and epithelial linings of the entire reproductive tract

    Also: a) Oviducts: increased motility and ciliary activity
          b) Uterus:   increased motility
                     secretion of abundant, clear cervical mucus
          c) Vagina:   increased "cornification" (layering of epithelial cells)

3. Growth of external genitalia
4. Growth of breasts (particularly ducts)
5. Development of female body configuration: narrow shoulders, broad hips, converging thighs, diverging arms
6. Stimulation of fluid sebaceous gland secretions ("anti-acne")
7. Pattern of pubic hair (actual growth of pubic and axillary hair is androgen-stimulated)
8. Stimulation of protein anabolism and closure of the epiphyses (? due to stimulation of adrenal androgens)
9. Sex drive and behavior (? role of androgens)
10. Reduction of blood cholesterol
11. Vascular effects (deficiency $\longrightarrow$ "hot flashes")
12. Feedback effects on hypothalamus and anterior pituitary

---

Effects of progesterone

---

1. Stimulation of secretion by endometrium; also induces thick, sticky cervical secretions
2. Stimulation of growth of myometrium (in pregnancy)
3. Decrease in motility of oviducts and uterus
4. Decrease in vaginal "cornification"
5. Stimulation of breast growth (particularly glandular tissue)
6. Inhibition of effects of prolactin on the breasts
7. Elevation of body temperature
8. Feedback effects on hypothalamus and anterior pituitary

---

*After: Vander, H. J., et al. *Human Physiology* (New York: McGraw-Hill, 1975), p. 447.

## Accessory Organs

Oviducts

The **oviducts**, also called the uterine (or Fallopian) tubes, are about 4 inches long and extend from the uterus to the ovaries (fig. 8.2). These muscular tubes are lined by cells possessing **cilia**, little hairlike structures that beat toward the uterus. The tubes are not at all attached to the ovaries and instead have fingerlike projections called fimbria that sweep over the ovary at the time of ovulation. When the egg bursts from the ovary during ovulation, it is usually sucked up into an oviduct by the combined action of these projections and the beating of the cilia. Since only one egg is produced a month, it is believed by some that the ovaries take turns ovulating. More than one ovulation and subsequent fertilization explains the phenomenon of fraternal twins. Fraternal twins share a common father but are derived from different zygotes.

Since an egg must traverse a small space before entering an oviduct, it can possibly get lost and enter the abdominal cavity. Such eggs usually disintegrate but rarely have been fertilized in the abdominal cavity and even more rarely have come to term, the child being delivered by surgery. Development of a zygote anywhere outside the uterus is called an **ectopic pregnancy**.

Once in the oviduct, the egg is at first propelled rapidly by cilia movement and tubular muscle contraction. Soon the contractions diminish and the egg moves more slowly toward the uterus. Fertilization usually occurs in an oviduct because the egg lives only approximately 6 to 24 hours. Following fertilization, the developing zygote normally arrives at the uterus after several days and then **embeds** itself in the uterine lining, which has been prepared to receive it. Occasionally, the zygote becomes embedded into the wall of an oviduct where it begins to develop. Tubular pregnancies cannot succeed because the tubes are not anatomically capable of allowing full development to occur.

Uterus

The single **uterus** is about the size and shape of an inverted pear and lies tipped forward over the urinary bladder between the bladder and the rectum (fig. 8.1). The organ is held in place by ligaments called the uterine ligaments, but even so its position changes according to the fullness of the bladder and rectum (fig. 8.6). If the bladder is full, the uterus is moved backward; if the rectum is full, the uterus is moved more forward.

The muscular uterus has three portions (fig. 8.2)—the fundus, the body, and the cervix. The oviducts join the uterus just below the fundus and the **cervix** enters into the vagina at a nearly right angle. The opening of the cervix, called the os, leads to the vaginal canal.

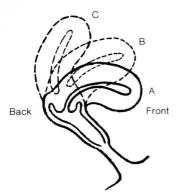

C

B

A

Back     Front

Figure 8.6   Approximate location of uterus in standing woman
(a) bladder and rectum empty, (b) bladder and rectum full,
(c) full bladder and empty rectum. (After Goldstein, *Human
Sexuality*, McGraw Hill, 1975.)

Menstrual Cycle—Non-Pregnant

| | F.S.H. | |
| | Estrogen | |
| | L.H. | |
| | Progesterone | |

| Follicle and Corpus Luteum | |
| Endometrium | |
| Myometrium | |

| Phases | Menstrual | Proliferation | Secretory | | Menstrual |
|---|---|---|---|---|---|
| Week | 1st | 2nd | 3rd | 4th | 1st |

Figure 8.7   Menstrual cycle showing the varying levels of
hormones that accompany the ovarian and menstrual cycles.
(Source: Courtesy of Ward's Natural Science Establishment,
Inc.)

Development of the embryo takes place in the uterus. This organ, sometimes called the womb, is capable of stretching to over twelve inches to accommodate the growing baby. The lining, called the **endometrium**, participates in the formation of the **placenta** (p. 159), which supplies the nutrients needed for embryonic and fetal development.

The endometrium has two layers: a basal layer and an inner functional layer. The functional layer of the endometrium varies in thickness according to a monthly cycle, called the **menstrual cycle**. The menstrual cycle is controlled principally by the ovarian hormones, estrogen and progesterone. With increased production of estrogen by an ovarian follicle, the endometrium thickens, becoming vascular and glandular (fig. 8.7). This is called the **proliferation phase** of the menstrual cycle. With increased production of progesterone by the corpus luteum, the endometrium doubles in thickness and the uterine glands become mature, producing a thick, mucoid secretion rich in glycogen. This is called the **secretory phase** of the menstrual cycle. The endometrium is now prepared to receive the developing zygote, which usually becomes embedded in the lining several days following fertilization. During this process, called **implantation**, the developing zygote becomes enclosed by the uterine lining where development continues.

If implantation does not occur, the corpus luteum begins to degenerate, progesterone level decreases, and the functional layer of the endometrium breaks down. Blood, cells, and glandular secretions flow from the uterus as the thickened layer is shed. This phase of the menstrual cycle is called the **menstrual flow** (or **menstruation**, or **the menses**). Menstrual flow results in a discharge of 1 to 6 ounces. Before menstruation has completely ceased, repair begins under the influence of estrogen from the ovary where follicular development is again underway.

*The menstrual and ovarian cycles.* The menstrual and ovarian cycles are synchronized because both are ultimately under the control of the anterior pituitary hormones FSH and LH. Figure 8.7 and chart 8.3 indicate how the ovarian cycle brings about the menstrual cycle. Day one of each cycle is taken to be the first day of the menses. While menstruation is occuring, a new follicle is being developed in the ovaries, therefore, repair of the endometrium begins even as menstruation is ceasing. Following ovulation, production of progesterone by the corpus luteum prepares the uterine lining to receive the zygote. If fertilization has not occurred or if the zygote is unable to implant itself, the corupus luteum degenerates and the uterine lining breaks down.

**Chart 8.3**
Ovarian and Menstrual Cycles

| Ovarian Cycle Phases | Events | Menstrual Cycle Phases | Events |
|---|---|---|---|
| Follicular<br><br>Days 1–13 | FSH<br><br>Follicle Maturation<br><br>Estrogen | Menstruation Days 1–5 | Endometrium breaks down |
| | | Proliferation Days 6–13 | Endometrium rebuilds |

O V U L A T I O N    Day 14˙

| Luteal<br><br>Days 15–28 | LH<br><br>Corpus Luteum<br><br>Progesterone | Secretory<br><br>Days 15–28 | Endometrium thickens and glands secrete glycogen |
|---|---|---|---|

˙Assuming a 28-day cycle.

Some people believe that women experience mood changes according to the level of sex hormones and the corresponding time of the monthly cycle. Low estrogen levels in particular have been associated with such emotions as anxiety, tension, depression, and irritability, while high estrogen levels have been associated with confidence and cheerfulness. So many factors affect mood that studies in this regard have not been decisive.

*Menarche and menopause.*    The **menarche** is the first menstrual cycle and **menopause** is the cessation of the menstrual cycle. Menopause is likely to occur between the ages of forty-five and fifty-five. As menopause develops, the menstrual cycles become irregular, but as long as they occur it is still possible for a woman to conceive and become pregnant. Therefore, a woman is usually not considered to have completed menopause until there has been no menstruation for a year. Menopause is associated with certain physical symptoms such as "hot flashes," which are caused by circulatory irregularities; dizziness; headaches; insomnia; sleepiness; and depression. Again, there is a great variation between women and any of these symptoms may be absent altogether.

Women sometimes report an increased sex drive following menopause and it has been suggested that this may be due to androgen production by the adrenal cortex or even by the ovaries themselves.

## Vagina

The vagina is a 5- to 6-inch muscular tube that makes a 45° angle with the small of the back (fig. 8.1). The lining of the vagina lies in folds called rugae, which are capable of extension as the muscular wall stretches. This capacity to extend is especially important when the vagina serves as the birth canal, and it may facilitate intercourse when the vagina receives the penis during copulation.

Glycogen produced by cells in the lining of the vagina is metabolized to acids inside the vagina. These acids are believed to prevent bacterial infections of the genital tract. But it also makes the vagina hostile to sperm because sperm prefer an alkaline rather than an acid medium. Since seminal fluid is alkaline, it is capable of neutralizing the vagina.

## Ovulation

Sometimes women would like to know the day of ovulation in order to increase their chances of becoming pregnant. Ovulation usually occurs on the fourteenth day prior to the first day of the next menstrual bleeding. This is not terribly helpful information, because it is generally not known ahead of time just when the first day of the next bleeding will be.

Methods for determining ovulation that are based on the differing effects of estrogen and progesterone have been discovered. Just prior to ovulation, estrogenic effects are apt to be most pronounced; after ovulation, progesterone effects are apt to be pronounced. Both of these hormones affect the mucus secreted by the cervix. Under the influence of estrogen, the mucus is abundant, clear, and nonviscous, especially just before ovulation. In contrast, progesterone causes the cervical mucus to become thick and sticky so that it forms a plug. High estrogen levels also cause a degree of cornification, or hardening, of sloughed off vaginal cells. Microscopic examination of vaginal cells by a physician can possibly indicate when and if ovulation is taking place. Progesterone causes body temperature to rise almost immediately following ovulation; therefore, the basal (or resting) temperature may be taken each morning prior to rising to try to determine if ovulation has occurred (fig. 8.8).

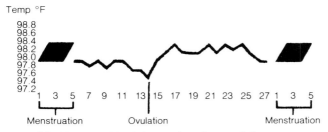

Figure 8.8   Typical oral body temperature changes during a 28-day menstrual cycle.

Since all of these methods for determining the time of ovulation are rather imprecise, they are usually more helpful when a woman is trying to become pregnant than when she is trying to prevent pregnancy.

## External Genitals

The external genital organs of the female (fig. 8.9) are known collectively as the **vulva**. The **mons pubis**, a fatty prominence underlying the pubic hair, may be included in this category because it has some sexual significance, being highly sensitive due to its many touch receptors. The **labia majora**, two large folds of skin that extend backward from the mons pubis on either side, mark the outer boundaries of the vulva. The outer sides of the labia majora are pigmented and have hair, but the inner sides are smooth and have numerous modified sweat glands. Since the labia majora develops from embryonic genital folds as does the scrotum, they are considered homologous to the scrotum.

The **labia minora** are two small folds lying just inside the labia majora. They consist of smooth, pigmented skin and extend upward from the vaginal opening to encircle and form a foreskin for the **clitoris**, an organ that is homologous to the penis. Although quite small, the clitoris has a shaft of erectile tissue and is capped by a pea-shaped glans. The clitoris also has receptors that allow it to function as a sexually sensitive organ.

The **vestibule**, a cleft between the labia minora, contains the openings of the urethra and the vagina. The urethra is part of the urinary system, while the vagina is the copulatory organ of females. Notice then that the urinary system and the reproductive system are separate in the female. The vagina may be

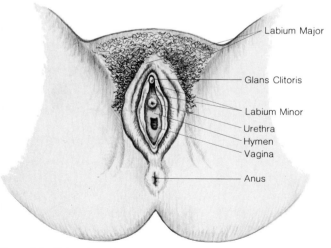

Figure 8.9   External genitalia of the female.

Human Reproduction

partially closed by a ring of tissue called the **hymen**. The hymen may persist or be disrupted by all types of physical activities, not necessarily sexual intercourse; therefore, its presence or absence should not be associated with virginity or lack of it.

## Summary

The female gonads are the ovaries that are located one on each side of the upper pelvic cavity. Inside the ovaries are numerous follicles. Each month one follicle matures completely producing estrogen and an egg, which bursts from the ovary during ovulation. Then, the follicle becomes the corpus luteum that produces the other female sex hormone, progesterone. Estrogen causes the uterine lining (endometrium) to build up and progesterone causes the uterine lining to become secretory. The egg usually enters one of the two oviducts that lead to the uterus. The egg is fertilized within the oviduct before proceeding to the uterus where the developing zygote implants itself in the endometrium lining.

If fertilization does not occur, the endometrium is shed during the menses. The ovarian (and menstrual cycle) has two parts: the follicular (proliferation) phase is under the control of the anterior pituitary hormone, FSH, which promotes maturation of a follicle and the luteal (secretory) phase is under the control of LH, which maintains the corpus luteum. Feedback control can explain the occurrence of the two phases including menstruation.

## Terms

| | |
|---|---|
| clitoris | mons pubis |
| endometrium | oocyte |
| follicular phase | ovarian cycle |
| implantation | ovarian follicle |
| labia majora | oviducts |
| labia minora | ovulation |
| luteal phase | proliferation phase |
| menarche | secretory phase |
| menopause | uterus |
| menses | vagina |
| menstrual cycle | |

## Review

1. Describe the events of the ovarian cycle and state the hormones associated with each event.
2. Describe the accessory organs and state the function of each.
3. Describe how the events of the menstrual cycle are related to the events of the ovarian cycle.
4. Name the external genitals of the female and state their anatomical position in relation to each other.

# Human Sexuality

9

Human sexuality may be seen as encompassing three aspects: gender identity, gender role, and sexual conduct (fig. 9.1). **Gender identity** is one's self-concept, that is, the self-perception we have of ourself as a girl or boy or a woman or man. Usually, this self-concept is related to the sex organs; in other words, persons born with male genitals come to think of themselves as men, while persons born with female genitals come to think of themselves as women. Occasionally, there are variations, however.

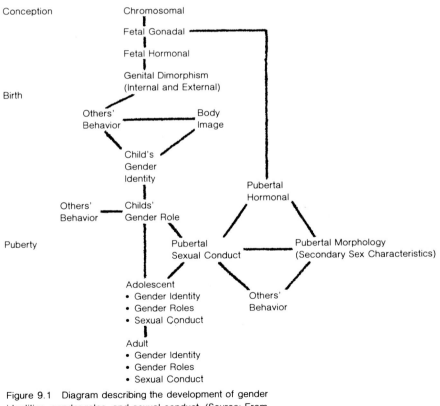

Figure 9.1  Diagram describing the development of gender identities, gender roles, and sexual conduct. (Source: From *Human Sexualities* by John H. Gagnon. Copyright © 1977 by Scott, Foresman, and Company. Reprinted by permission.)

**Gender role** refers to the behavior that is commonly accepted as appropriate to a girl or boy or a woman or man. Gender roles are being questioned recently, but there are some toys and play activities that many people still specifically associate with girls or with boys. And in spite of recent attitude shifts, there is often a dichotomy of responsibilities in adult life; certain responsibilities or roles are often assumed by a woman and certain other responsibilities are often assumed by a man.

**Sexual conduct** means the manner in which one satisfies the sex drive. The sex drive is not like other biological drives such as those having to do with eating and sleeping. These drives must be satisfied or death follows. The sex drive varies greatly in intensity and does not have to be satisfied at all. Therefore, a person can have a gender identity and gender role appropriate to his/her sex but still not engage in sexual activities.

There has been much discussion about whether gender identity, gender role, and sexual conduct are determined by biological or environmental factors. As figure 9.1 indicates, the chromosomes direct the eventual formation of the fetal gonads and these in turn produce sex hormones so that we are eventually born either a girl or boy. However, knowing that we are a girl or boy must be learned. And not only do the people around us teach us that we are male or female, they are also inclined to teach us what is appropriate behavior for males and females. Thus, it is often said that an interaction between biological and environmental factors shapes the way we think and behave. In figure 9.1 the actions of others are indicated as being important to the child's realization of gender identity and gender role.

There are those who believe that biological makeup is important only in that we are born either a girl or boy and that thereafter gender identity and gender role are learned. Gagnon expresses this position in the following manner:

Since there is no "natural" relationship between gender identity and gender-role performances, the child possesses a label with very little content. The label has a forward function, that is, it is used to organize the new things that happen. This is done by observing who works to earn the principal income, who is in charge of the housework, and who plays with cars or dolls. All of these activities are more or less gender typed, mostly by frequency rather than dramatic differences, and by verbal exhortations of what boys do and what girls do.[1]

Figure 9.1 indicates that the gender identity of childhood is reinforced at the time of puberty, when the secondary sex characteristics appear. By this time also, gender roles taught by society may be clearly understood (fig. 9.2). The sexual behavior that usually begins at the time of adolescence is dependent to a degree on gender identity and gender role. Since both of these have a biological component, sexual conduct has a biological component. Certainly, the anatomy

1. John H. Gagnon, *Human Sexualities* (Glenview, Ill.: Scott, Foresman & Co., 1977), p. 68.

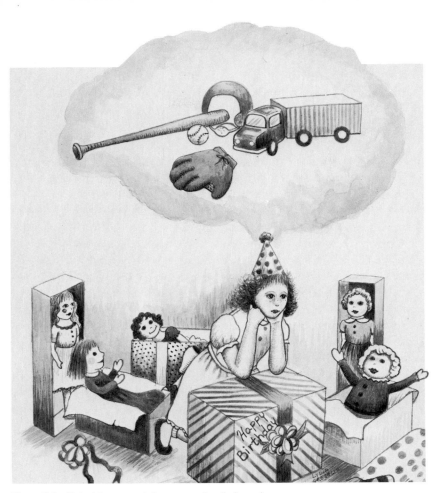

Figure 9.2 Pictorial representation suggesting that gender roles are encouraged by society.

of our bodies determines to a degree how we will act sexually. But within these prescribed limits, sexual conduct may be largely learned. In figure 9.1 the adult's gender identity, gender role, and sexual conduct is seen as an outgrowth of the adolescent's gender identity, gender role, and sexual conduct.

In chapter 15, we will be presenting circumstantial evidence to suggest that genes might possibly influence the manner in which we act out our adult reproductive gender roles. This is not meant to negate the fact that humans do learn much of their behavior. As a matter of fact, humans could even learn to ignore inclinations that might be generated by possessing certain genes. Therefore, if there is a genetic difference between men and women such that men are more apt to seek a career and women are more apt to stay at home, this does not mean that gender roles could not change as society changes. It simply means that there might be a certain amount of resistance to change due to our biological makeup rather than a purely psychological resistance to change.

## Gender Identity and Role

In our society, traditionally persons with male genitals who have a *masculine gender identity* and accept the *masculine gender role* usually have a heterosexual relationship (i.e., a relationship with the opposite sex) that includes being married and assuming financial responsibility for a wife and children. Traditionally, persons with female genitals who have a *feminine gender identity* and accept the *female gender role* usually have a heterosexual relationship that includes being married and taking care of a husband, children, and a home. Within this framework, the male is often envisioned as being more competent and aggressive, while the female is envisioned as being more submissive and gentle. Sexual prowess is more important in the male, while physical attractiveness is more important in the female.

There are more variations in sex roles today than there have ever been before in our society. Therefore, it is not unusual to find individuals and couples who do not act out the accepted sex roles and who have developed sex role patterns more suitable to their own circumstances. Sometimes both sexes work and share in the duties of the household and children. Sometimes, men and women live together without being married and without having children. In other instances, a man may stay at home and take care of the house and children while the woman works. Also, homosexual men live together and lesbian women live together, forming stable and lasting relationships. If so, they might provide a home for adopted children or children of former heterosexual marriages.

### Gender Identity and Gender Role Conflicts

There are some persons who have the genitals of one sex but prefer the sex role and sexual conduct of the opposite sex. Males feel that they are women trapped in a man's body, and females feel that they are men trapped in a woman's body.

These persons are called **transsexuals**, and they may decide to undergo a sex change operation. The proper hormonal treatment along with supplemental operative procedures to alter the shape of the larynx, breasts, and hips can bring about development of the secondary sex characteristics. In males, the penis and scrotum can be removed and a vagina constructed. In females, a scrotum can be formed from labial tissues and a penis can be constructed from the clitoris plus skin grafts. However, this manufactured penis is incapable of an erection. Photographs of persons who have had their sex changed testify to how well these individuals can assume the outward appearance of their new sex.

Some persons feel that they are both male and female and so they like to cross-dress in order to express the other side of their nature. Sometimes these persons have both a male and female name and function in two different settings; in one setting they play a male role and in the other setting they play a female role. Persons who want to retain their present genitals but who like to cross-dress are called **transvestites**. They may be homosexuals, but most are heterosexuals.

## Sexual Conduct

Sexual conduct will be considered to have two aspects: (1) the selection of a partner and (2) sexual activities with the partner.

Sexual Partner

One can achieve sexual stimulation and orgasm without a partner (p. 137) but in many instances sex partners stimulate each other. Most adults choose other adults for their partners.

*Consenting Adult Relationships.* A heterosexual relationship is one in which a man and woman engage in foreplay and sexual intercourse. This is the most common type of sexual relationship in our society. The man and woman may be married to each other; single; planning to be married; not planning to be married; or already married to someone else.

Gay men and women have homosexual relationships with other men and women respectively. Homosexuals do not necessarily have a gender identity and a gender role conflict. A man may very well identify himself as a man and prefer a man's gender role but still want to relate sexually to another man. Lesbians, too, are apt to identify themselves as women and may prefer a woman's gender role.

Bisexuals are individuals who are involved in both heterosexual and homosexual relationships. They may be married to a member of the opposite sex and engage in homosexual activities outside the home or they may be single and alternately engage in heterosexual and homosexual relationships.

There is evidence to suggest that there is often no clear-cut dichotomy between heterosexuality and homosexuality, meaning that many persons are bisexual to a degree. In 1972, the Playboy Foundation sponsored a nationwide investigation of sexual attitudes and behavior of over 2,000 American adults from various parts of the country. One of the questions designed by the investigator Morton Hunt was, "Is there some homosexuality in all of us?" Roughly half of the sample felt this was true.[2] The Institute for Sex Research at Indiana University found that men who frequented gay bars did not always choose male partners (chart 9.1).

2. M. Hunt, *Sexual Behavior in the 1970s* (Chicago: Playboy Press, 1974).

## Chart 9.1

Percentage of Respondents from Gay Bars and Organizations Stating Sexual Preferences

| | |
|---|---|
| Exclusively homosexual | 50.6 |
| Predominantly homosexual, only insignificantly heterosexual | 29.8 |
| Predominantly homosexual, but significantly heterosexual | 13.1 |
| Equally homosexual and heterosexual | 4.4 |
| Predominantly heterosexual, but significantly homosexual | 2.1 |

N  =  1,057

From *Male Homosexuals: Their Problems and Adaptations*, p. 112, by Weinberg, Martin S. and Williams, Colin J. Copyright © 1974 by Oxford University Press, Inc. Reprinted by permission.

*Other types of relationships.*   Some persons called **prostitutes** become willing sex partners if they are paid. In most cases, a man is paying for the services of a female or another male. Prostitutes who solicit work by walking the streets are called **"streetwalkers."** Female streetwalkers often turn over their pay to a man, called a pimp, who may be both a sex partner and an agent. Female prostitutes can also work in "whorehouses" or in massage parlors, or they may be "call girls," serving their clients either in their own apartments or in the clients' residences. Male prositutes may solicit work in public places or they may be kept by an older man who employs them under the guise of some other position, such as a private secretary or chauffeur.

**Rape** is defined variously in state statutes but usually takes the form of penile-vaginal contact; oral-genital contact; or sodomy, penile-anal contact, without consent. *Statutory rape* is having sexual contact with a young person (for example, less than age sixteen) even if consent has been given. In most instances, males rape females or other males. *Gang rapes* occur when a number of individuals subdue a single victim. *Forcible rape* is the use of violence or the threat of violence to cause submission.

Paul Gebhard and his colleagues categorize rapists as being one of five types. There are those who are hostile and assaultive, those who are amoral delinquents, those who commit rape only as part of a drunken episode, those who suddenly and surprisingly engage in an explosive attack, and those who only force themselves on "the kind of girl who is asking for it."[3]

**Incest** is sexual relations between individuals who are so closely related that they would not be able to marry legally. About 15 percent of the people surveyed by Morton Hunt said that they had had sexual contact with relatives, but only 7 percent admitted to coitus (sexual intercourse) with relatives.[4] This occurred mostly between siblings or between cousins.

3. P. H. Gebhard et al., *Sex Offenders: An Analysis of Types* (New York: Harper-Hoeber, 1965).
4. M. Hunt, *Sexual Behavior in the 1970s* (Chicago: Playboy Press, 1974).

**Pedophilia** is the use of children for sexual gratification. In some cases, the adult is related to the child and so the situation goes unnoticed by the law, but in other instances the adult is charged with child molesting. While most people tend to think that child molesters are homosexuals, this is not necessarily the case and they are just as likely to be heterosexuals.

**Gerontophilia** is the use of old people for sexual purposes, and **necrophilia** is the desire to have sex with dead people. In these cases, the possibility of resistance is minimal and nil.

Both males and females have been reported to have sexual contact with animals, which is called **bestiality**. A. C. Kinsey, who interviewed 5,300 males and 5,490 females in the late 1940s found that 17 percent of male adolescents who lived on farms had sexual contact to orgasm with animals. Urban males, who have less opportunity, reported about 8 percent contact with animals. According to this data, females are less likely to engage in erotic activities with animals; the reported incidence was only about 4 percent.

Indirect Sex

Some individuals who do not form sexual relationships with other individuals rely on indirect sexual experiences for sexual gratification. For example, **fetishism** is sexual stimulation derived from an inanimate object. The object is sometimes used to assist the attainment of orgasm during self-stimulation. Fetishism can also include sexual stimulation derived from parts of the body not usually considered sexual, such as feet, hair, limbs, and hands. In this case, the fetish can assist the attainment of sexual stimulation prior to sexual intercourse. **Voyeurism** is receiving sexual gratification from seeing someone in the nude or watching sexual intercourse. Most people can be stimulated by voyeurism, but they do not actively try to peek at others as "peeping Toms" do. This type of voyeurism is a misdemeanor.

Obscene phone calls are a form of indirect sex; the caller is stimulated by the shock and dismay of the victim. The same may be said for the **exhibitionist** who displays his/her genitals suddenly to innocent bystanders. Reacting coolly and disinterested in both instances can thwart the person's desired effect. In the case of an obscene phone call, it is wise to end the conversation immediately after the first obscene remark.

**Pornography** is the use of visual or written materials to cause sexual arousal. Pornography is more accepted today than before. Pornographic literature and films are readily available and are not subject to stringent censorship.

Chart 9.2 lists sexual behaviors that are sometimes considered to be sexual offenses and indicates the effectiveness of legal control.

# Chart 9.2

Classifications of Sexual Offenses

| | Types of Sexual Conduct | Legal Labels | Incidences in the Population |
|---|---|---|---|
| **Heterosexual** | | | |
| Conventional | 1) Pre-marital sex<br>  (1) Between youths and<br>  (2) Between adults and<br>      youths (victim?) | Sex delinquency, incorrigibility contributing to delinquency, statutory rape | Common |
| | 2) Pre-marital, post-marital, extra-marital sex | Fornication, cohabitation, adultery | Very common |
| | 3) Sex techniques | Sodomy, crimes against nature | Very common |
| | 4) Female prostitution | Prostitution, soliciting, loitering, disorderly conduct | Many consumers, few sellers |
| | 5) Pornography | Obscenity, pornography | Many consumers |
| | 6) Forced sex<br>  adults (victim)<br>  youth (victim) | Rape, indecent assault, attempted rape | Somewhat common |
| | 7) Voyeurism (victim) | Voyeurism | Uncommon |
| | 8) Exhibitionism (victim) | Exhibitionism | |
| | 9) Sex with children (victim) | Child molesting, lewd and lascivious, indecent assault, sodomy | to |
| | 10) Incest<br>  child and youth (victim)<br>  adult (victim?) | Incest, and all of 9 above | |
| | 11) Forced sex<br>  children (victim) | Rape, see 6 | Very rare |
| **Homosexual** | 12) With adults | Crime against nature, lewd conduct, sodomy, soliciting | Fairly common |
| | Youth (victim) | See 9, 1 | Somewhat common |
| | Children (victim) | See 9 | Uncommon |
| | 13) Male prostitution | Sodomy, see 4 | Somewhat common |
| | 14) Pornography | See 5 | Many customers |
| **Animal contacts** | 15) Animal contacts | Bestiality, crime against nature, sodomy | Rare |

| Proportion of Events Reported to Police | Police Activity | Effectiveness of Legal Control on Rates of Behavior |
| --- | --- | --- |
| Rare | (1) Only against sexually active young women<br>(2) Some older males arrested | Nil |
| Nil | Extremely rare, usually for non-sexual reasons | Nil |
| Nil | Harassment, particular circumstances | |
| Rare—by moral entrepreneurs, not participants | Sporadic campaigns, keeping public order, often involves police corruption | Low could be effective due to public nature of offenses |
| Rare—by moral entrepreneurs, not participants | Sporadic campaigns, now limited by court decisions | Low |
| Some | Limited by sexism, often unresponsive to victims | Low could be somewhat more effective |
| Few | Minimum reaction to reports, unlikely to make arrest | Very low |
| Few to some | Minimum reaction unless children are involved | Low |
| Few to some | React strongly to reports | Low |
| Few | React to reports, particularly with children | Low |
| Many | Very strong reaction | |
| | Sporadic campaign, harassment | Low could be more effective |
| Few/few some | | |
| See 4 | Strong reaction to reports | |
| See 5 | | |
| Nil | May react to report | Nil |

## Sexual Activities

Sexual conduct not only includes choosing a partner, it also includes sexual activities. Chart 9.3 lists various activities that investigator James Curran thought might be experienced by young heterosexual people. (Actually, however, homosexuals can engage in these same activities as long as anatomy permits.) The subjects were eighty-eight male and seventy-six female students from a large, relatively conservative, midwestern university. The chart shows the percentages of males and females who answered "yes" to the twenty-one items. Comparison shows that there is no double standard as far as these young people are concerned; in fact, beginning with item number 9 an approximately equal or even greater number of females than males indicated that they experienced the types of sexual behavior stated.

Several items are worthy of discussion. **Foreplay** includes all those physical activitites that sexually arouse a partner prior to **intercourse**, which is most often the act of having the penis in the vagina. In regard to chart 9.3, foreplay could include all items but numbers 11 and 19. Foreplay involves the stimulation

**Chart 9.3**
Percentage of Yes Responses to Heterosexual Behavior Scale

| Have you ever engaged in the following behavior with a member of the opposite sex? | Percentage of Males Saying "Yes" | Percentage of Females Saying "Yes" |
|---|---|---|
| 1. One minute of continuous kissing on the lips? | 86.4 | 89.2 |
| 2. Manual manipulation of clothed female breasts? | 82.7 | 71.1 |
| 3. Manual manipulation of bare female breasts? | 75.5 | 66.3 |
| 4. Manual manipulation of clothed female genitals? | 76.4 | 67.5 |
| 5. Kissing nipples of female breast? | 65.5 | 59.0 |
| 6. Manual manipulation of bare female genitals? | 64.4 | 60.2 |
| 7. Manual manipulation of clothed male genitals? | 57.3 | 51.8 |
| 8. Mutual manipulation of genitals? | 55.5 | 50.6 |
| 9. Manual manipulation of bare male genitals? | 50.0 | 51.8 |
| 10. Manual manipulation of female genitals until there were massive secretions? | 49.1 | 50.6 |
| 11. Sexual intercourse, face to face? | 43.6 | 37.3 |
| 12. Manual manipulation of male genitals to ejaculation? | 37.3 | 41.0 |
| 13. Oral contact with female genitals? | 31.8 | 42.2 |
| 14. Oral contact with male genitals? | 30.9 | 42.2 |
| 15. Mutual manual manipulation of genitals to mutual orgasm? | 30.9 | 26.5 |
| 16. Oral manipulation of male genitals? | 30.0 | 38.6 |
| 17. Oral manipulation of female genitals? | 30.0 | 41.0 |
| 18. Mutual oral-genital manipulation? | 20.9 | 28.9 |
| 19. Sexual intercourse, entry from the rear? | 14.5 | 22.9 |
| 20. Oral manipulation of male genitals to ejaculation? | 22.7 | 26.5 |
| 21. Mutual oral manipulation of genitals to mutual orgasm? | 13.6 | 12.0 |

Curran, J. P. Convergance toward a single sexual standard? *Social Behavior and Personality.*

of **erogenous** zones, areas of the body where there is a concentration of nerve endings and areas that the person associates with sexual arousal.

Oral-genital manipulation occurs when one partner stimulates the genitals of the other by using the mouth and tongue. **Cunnilingus** involves kissing, tonguing, and sucking the clitorus and labial structures, while **fellatio** involves licking and sucking the penis.

Mutual manipulation of the genitals would be a form of masturbation. **Masturbation** is also self-stimulation of the genitals and other erogenous zones. In a study of college students in the New York City area, 89 percent of the males and 61 percent of the females reported that they masturbated themselves.[5] Some people believe that self-stimulation may be physically harmful, but the physical effects of masturbation are no different from the effects of any other sexual activity.

*Sadomasochism.*

Aside from the activities such as those listed in chart 9.3, there are two psychological problems that are often mentioned in regard to sexual conduct. A person who enjoys inflicting pain on another is called a **sadist**, and a person who enjoys receiving pain is a **masochist**. When a sadist has sexual contact with a masochist, the sadist may be sexually gratified when physically mistreating the masochistic partner and the masochist may be sexually gratified when being mistreated. While extreme sadomasochism may be rare, Morton Hunt found that a small percentage of males and females have obtained sexual pleasure in inflicting or receiving pain from biting, hitting, scratching, and pinching (chart 9.4).[6]

**Sexual intercourse**, also called *coitus* or *copulation*, usually refers to the heterosexual act of having the penis within the vagina. However, the term can be used to include **sodomy**, which is the act of having the penis in the anus. Sodomy can be a heterosexual event or a homosexual event between men.

There are numerous positions for sexual intercourse (fig. 9.3). Some positions are listed in chart 9.5 along with a few possible advantages and disadvantages for each. Choice of a position (or positions) could possibly be the result of experimentation or in some instances it could be the result of societal customs. There are those who argue that the vagina is so situated in humans that the man on top position is the easiest to maintain. There are others who argue that the man on top position is prevalent in socities where men are dominant and women are submissive. Of course, if couples use a number of different positions, the latter argument becomes less tenable.

5. S. Arafat and W. D. Cotton, "Masturbation Practices of Males and Females" *Journal of Sex Research* (New York: Society for the Scientific Study Sex, 1974).
6. Hunt, *Sexual Behavior in the 1970s.*

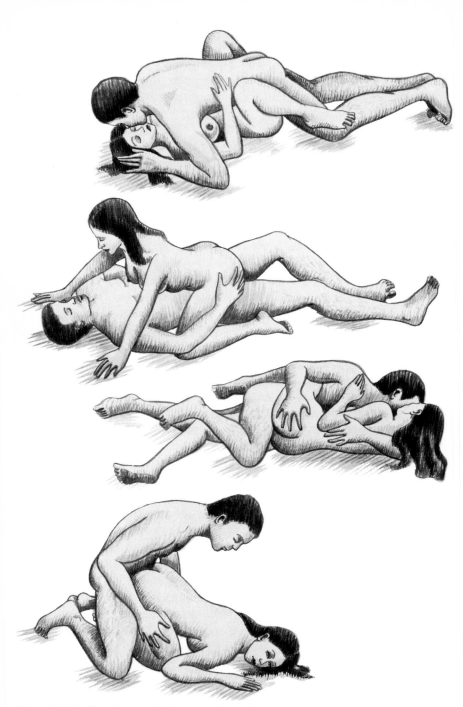

Figure 9.3   Positions for sexual intercourse: face to face, man
above, face to face, woman above, side by side, and rear
entry.

**Chart 9.4**

Ever Obtained Sexual Pleasure from Inflicting or Receiving Pain:
By Age and Sex, Total National Sample, Percents

|  | Males | | Females | |
|---|---|---|---|---|
|  | Under 35 | 35 and Over | Under 35 | 35 and Over |
| Inflicting pain | 6.2 | 2.9 | 2.5 | 1.5 |
| Receiving pain | 3.7 | 1.0 | 5.4 | 3.5 |

Reprinted by permission of Playboy Press. From *Sexual Behavior in the 1970's*, p. 334, by Morton Hunt. Copyright © 1974 by Morton Hunt.

**Chart 9.5**

Positions for Intercourse

|  | Advantages | Disadvantages |
|---|---|---|
| Face to face, man above | Ease of penetration<br>Freedom of movement for man | Woman lacks freedom of movement<br>Man may be heavy for woman |
| Face to face, woman above | Freedom of movement for woman<br>Easier for man to delay ejaculation | Man lacks freedom of movement<br>Penis may slip out |
| Face to face, side position | Freedom of movement for both<br>Ejaculation can be delayed | Penetration by penis is shallow |
| Rear entry | Deep penetration by penis<br>Man's hands are free | Less personal<br>Woman supports weight |

## Summary

Human sexuality has three aspects—gender identity, gender role, and sexual conduct. There is a difference of opinion at this time as to the degree these aspects are genetically or environmentally determined.

Gender identity and role have traditionally meant that the male agressively pursues a career while the female demurely stays at home to raise children. However, many variations in gender roles are seen today.

Transsexuals are individuals who wish to change their gender identity, and transvestites are individuals who like to cross-dress thereby assuming the opposite gender role to a certain degree.

Sexual conduct is assumed to have two aspects: selection of a partner and sexual activities. Consenting adults usually form sexual partnerships, but there are other possibilities such as prostitution, rape, incest, pedophilia, gerontophilia, and bestiality. Some persons rely partially or wholly on indirect sexual experiences including fetishism, voyeurism, exhibitionism, and pornography.

Although self-masturbation is fairly common, sexual activities between consenting adults usually consist of foreplay and sexual intercourse, which can utilize several positions.

---

## Terms

| | |
|---|---|
| bestiality | homosexual (lesbian) |
| bisexual | masochist |
| coitus, copulation | masturbation |
| courtship | necrophilia |
| cunnilingus | pedophilia |
| erogenous zone | prostitute |
| exhibitionist | rape |
| fellatio | sadist |
| fetishism | sexual intercourse |
| foreplay | sodomy |
| gender identity | transsexual |
| gender role | transvestite |
| gerontophilia | voyeurism |

---

## Review

1. Give evidence to support the contention that gender identity, gender role, and sexual conduct are learned.

2. Give evidence to support the contention that gender roles are not clear-cut in today's society.

3. Put the following statement in your own words:

   The predominant part of gender-identity differentiation receives program by way of social transmission from those responsible for the reconfirmation of the sex of assignment in the daily practices of rearing. Once differentiated, gender identity receives further confirmation from the hormonal changes of puberty, or lack of confirmation in instances of incongruous identity.[7]

4. What is the predominant feeling of persons who want a sex-change operation?

5. How do transsexuals differ from transvestites?

6. Argue the contention that homosexual men are not necessarily effeminate and that lesbian women are not necessarily masculine.

7. J. Money and A. Ehrhardt, Man and Woman, Boy and Girl
   (New York: New American Library,), p. 4.

7. If an adult is afraid to approach another adult with the intention of proposing sex, then what other type of partner might be chosen? What are the common means by which individuals receive indirect sexual stimulation?

8. Discuss who is at fault—the rapist or the person being raped. Then, discuss who is at fault—the burglar or the homeowner. Did you have the same position for each of these? If not, why not?

9. Give arguments in favor of and opposed to pornography.

10. Some state laws attempt to regulate sexual activities between consenting adults. Argue that these activities should or should not be subject to regulation.

# 10 Orgasm and Fertilization

Sexual arousal, including sexual intercourse, can lead to psychological and physical reactions known collectively as an **orgasm**, which is sometimes considered to be the climax of the sex act. In order to discuss these reactions more fully, it is necessary to describe the anatomy and physiology of the perineum.

## Perineum

The **perineum** is the diamond-shaped area at the lower end of the trunk between the thighs and buttocks of both males and females (fig. 10.1). The muscles of the perineum extend to the base of the penis in males and the external genitals of the female are located in this region.

Male

The penis contains three longitudinal masses of erectile tissue (fig. 10.2).Two of these, the **corpora cavernosa**, are located above the urethra and extend from the glans penis to the base of the penis where they are surrounded by fibers of the **ischiocavernosus muscle**. The other mass of erectile tissue, the **corpus spongiosum**, surrounds the urethra and ends in the bulbus penis, which is enclosed by the **bulbocavernosus muscle** (fig. 10.1).

*Erection.*    Erection of the penis (fig. 10.3) usually occurs when a male is sexually aroused. During an erection, the penis becomes wider, longer, and firmer. Erection depends on the amount of blood entering the erectile tissue of the penis. Normally, the amount of blood entering the erectile tissue by way of the arterioles is the same as the amount of blood leaving by way of the venules and the penis is flaccid. But when the penis becomes erect, more blood enters than leaves the erectile tissue and the erectile tissue becomes congested with blood. This is an example of **vasocongestion**, which, in general, is considered to be an important sexual response.

Erection is controlled by two portions of the central nervous system; sexual response centers are located in the cord and in the brain. When a man thinks sexual thoughts or has sexual dreams, nerve impulses travel from the brain to a center in the cord, which in turn emits nerve impulses that cause dilation of the arterioles leading to the erectile tissue. Conscious thought is not required for an erection, and stimulation of the penis alone can cause an erection. In this

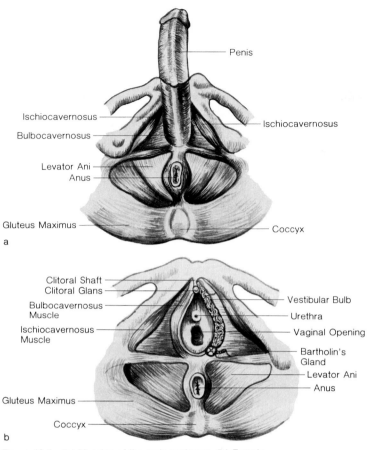

Figure 10.1 (a) Muscles of the male perineum. (b) Female perineum. Muscles have been removed from right side to reveal underlying structure.

case, erection occurs due to a simple reflex action in which touch receptors in the penis initiate nerve impulses that are received by the cord, and, thereafter, nerve impulses leaving the cord cause the arterioles to dilate and carry more blood. (Since an erection can occur automatically, it sometimes occurs unexpectedly.) Once the penis becomes erect, it may be introduced into the vagina of the female.

The scrotum also responds to sexual stimuli. Contraction of the muscles in the wall of the scrotum elevate the testes, which may have increased slightly in size.

*Ejacualtion.* Ejaculation has two phases: emission and expulsion. Emission has occurred when semen is present in the urethra. Expulsion has occurred when semen has been expelled from the urethra.

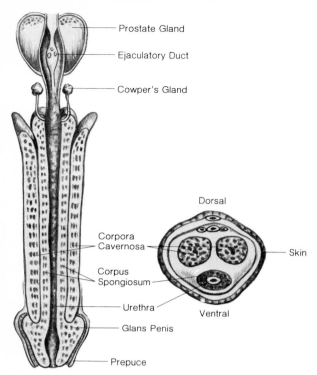

Figure 10.2   Longitudinal structure of penis and a cross section through the shaft of a penis.

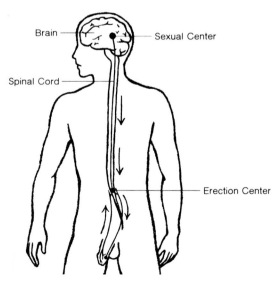

Figure 10.3   The nervous system initiates and controls erection. (After Goldstein, *Human Sexuality*, McGraw Hill, 1975.)

*Emission.* When sexual stimulation becomes intense the spinal cord sends nerve impulses via appropriate nerve fibers to the epididymides, ductus deferentia, and the ampullae. Their subsequent motility causes sperm to enter the urethra, whereupon the seminal vesicles, prostate gland, and Cowper's glands release their secretions. At this time, a small amount of the secretion from the Cowper's glands may leak from the end of the penis. Since this is a mucoid secretion, it has been suggested that this leakage may aid the process of intercourse by providing a certain amount of lubrication.

*Expulsion.* Filling of the urethra causes nerve impulses to be transmitted to the spinal cord. Subsequently, rhythmic nerve impulses from the cord cause rhythmical contractions of the ischiocavernosus and bulbocavernosus muscles and these contractions forcibly expel semen out of the urethra. The rhythmical contractions of the perineal muscles is an example of release from **myotonia**, or muscle tenseness. Myotonia is another important sexual response.

Following ejaculation, the penis, which became **tumescent**, or erect, now undergoes **detumescence** and becomes flaccid again. Some men experience a refractory period during which they cannot perform the sex act. The length of the refractory period varies with the individual and it is commonly believed to increase with age.

Female

In the female, the shaft of the *clitoris* contains erectile tissue homologous to the corpora cavernosa of the male. Corpus spongiosum-type tissue is found in the glans of the clitoris and the **vestibular bulbs** (fig. 10.1), which are located beneath the labia minora on each side of the vaginal opening. The **bulbocavernosus** muscle lies above the vestibular bulbs and surrounds the vaginal opening, forming a sphincter (circular muscle). The **levator ani muscles** surround the deeper parts of the vagina and when these muscles are constricted, the walls of the vagina are brought together.

Sexual response in the female may be more subtle than in the male, but it is possible to find corollaries. The clitoris is believed to be an especially sensitive organ for initiating sexual sensations. Nerve impulses from the clitoris, just like nerve impulses from the penis in males, enter the cord before being transmitted to the brain. It's possible too for the clitoris to become ever so slightly erect as the erectile tissue becomes engorged with blood. But vasocongestion is more obvious in the labia minora, which expand and deepen in color (fig. 10.4). Erectile tissue within the vaginal wall also expand with blood and the added pressure in these blood vessels causes small droplets of fluid to squeeze through the vessel walls and appear on the inner surface of the vagina. Another possible source of lubrication, especially in prolonged intercourse, is from the mucus-secreting **Bartholin's glands**, located beneath the labia minora on either side of the vagina.

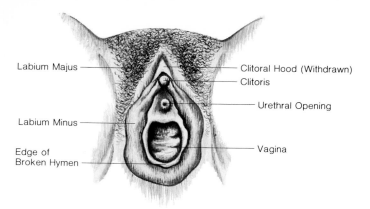

Labium Majus

Labium Minus

Edge of
Broken Hymen

Clitoral Hood (Withdrawn)

Clitoris

Urethral Opening

Vagina

Figure 10.4   Vasocongestion in the labia minora causes them
to expand as they deepen in color.

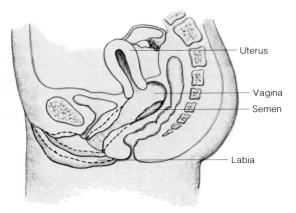

Uterus

Vagina
Semen

Labia

Figure 10.5   Sexual response in females includes a change in
the size and position of sexual organs. The uterus moves
backward as the vagina lengthens and expands to provide a
receptacle for semen. Myotonia causes the lower one-third of
the vagina to be constricted and vasocongestion causes the
labia minora to expand. Dottled lines show normal position of
vagina and labia.

During intercourse, the female pelvis is apt to move back and forth as the
penis thrusts in and out of the vagina. Contraction of the bulbocavernosus muscle
and the levator ani muscles can aid in having the vagina massage the penis.
It's possible for a woman to practice contracting the first of these muscles by
pretending to hold back urination and the second by pretending to prevent
defecation. Sometimes such practice is recommended for women who believe
that the vagina is not tight enough to provide adequate stimulation for the penis.
However, muscle contraction is reported to automatically constrict the lower one-
third of the vagina as the upper two-thirds of the vagina automatically lengthens

146                                        Human Reproduction

and distends to accommodate the penis. These changes in the vagina are believed to be accompanied by a shift in the position of the uterus (fig. 10.5).

Release from myotonia is especially evident in the female when the perineal muscles contract rhythmically, presumably as a result of nerve impulses from the spinal cord, just as rhythmical contractions of these muscles in the male are due to such impulses. It is also possible that nerve impulses from the cord increase uterine and oviduct motility and that this may assist the transport of sperm toward the tubes.

## Orgasm

*Orgasm*, which may be defined as reactions or sensations that occur at the climax of sexual stimulation, has both a physiological and psychological component. The psychological sensation of pleasure is centered in the brain, but the physiological reactions include not only those of the perineal region but of the whole body. The heart rate and blood pressure increase and there may be a flushing of the face and other parts of the body as blood rushes to the skin. *Vasocongestion* (engorgement by blood) occurs in specific regions. Breathing rate increases and *myotonia* (muscle tenseness) develops in various muscles.

Vasocongestion

Vasocongestion is apparent in the genitals of both sexes; for example, the penis becomes erect and the labia minora expand due to vasocongestion. Also, the breasts may swell (fig. 10.6) in women, and due to engorgement, the nipples may become erect in both men and women.

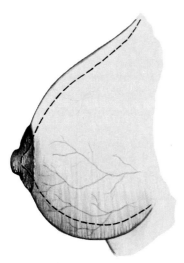

Figure 10.6  Vasocongestion in breast and nipple erection. Dotted lines show normal size.

Myotonia

Myotonia is apt to occur not only in the muscles about and near the genitals but also in the face, neck, limbs, abdomen, and buttocks. There may be an involuntary clutching of the partner due to contraction of the muscles in the fingers. Rhythmical contractions of the perineal muscles and possibly of the genitals themselves may be obvious signs that orgasm has occurred. This is especially true in the male because ejaculation due to rhythmical muscle contraction accompanies orgasm. Contraction signaling release from myotonia may be related to the sensation of orgasmic pleasure in the brain.

## Sexual Response

Investigation into human sexual responses has intensified during the past several years. Data are accumulating that may eventually enable a complete description of human sexual responses. In the meantime, the work of William H. Masters and Virginia E. Johnson has been reported widely. For the sake of describing sexual response in detail, these investigators divided sexual response into four phases: (1) **excitement phase**, (2) **plateau phase**, (3) **orgasmic phase**, and (4) **resolution phase**. The events that could possibly be associated with each of these phases are given in chart 10.1. It is important to realize that sexual

**Chart 10.1**
Phases in Sexual Response

| Male | Female |
|---|---|
| *Excitement Phase* | |
| Erection of the penis resulting from increased blood flow (vasocongestion). Penis increases in length and diameter. Partial elevation of testes and increase in size. | Moistening of vagina by appearance of beads of moisture on inner surface. Increase in size of clitoris. Elevation of uterus. |
| *Plateau Phase* | |
| Increase in circumference of glans penis. Full elevation of testes. Appearance at tip of penis of mucoid material from bulbourethral glands. (Cowper's glands) | Engorgement and swelling of tissues in outer third of vagina (orgasmic platform) and major labia. Ballooning of inner two-thirds of vagina. Further elevation of uterus and cervix. Enlargement of uterus; elevation of clitoris. Appearance of mucoid material from glands of Bartholin. |
| *Orgasmic Phase (Orgasm)* | |
| Ejaculation of semen resulting from contractions of the ductus (vas) deferens and accessory organs. Contraction of anal and urethral sphincters. | Contraction of uterus, orgasmic platform, anal and urethral sphincters. (Nothing in the nature of an ejaculation occurs.) |
| *Resolution Phase* | |
| Reduction in vasocongestion. Loss of penile erection. Refractory period sets in (i.e., inability to have another orgasm). May last for a few minutes or hours. | Reduction in vasocongestion. Reduction in orgasmic platform. Decrease in size of clitoris. Lack of a refractory period with ready return to orgasm. |

Source: *Human Sex and Sexuality* by Edwin B. Steen and James H. Price.

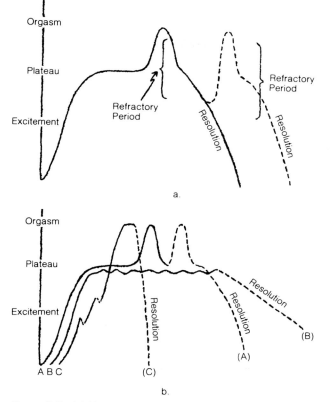

Figure 10.7 (a) Male sexual response and (b) female sexual response according to Masters and Johnson.

response is ongoing and has arbitrarily been divided into these four phases. Also, the phase descriptions pertain to events that are believed to occur generally, and individual differences are to be expected. The same may be said for the sexual response diagrams drawn by Masters and Johnson (fig. 10.7). The diagrams suggest that there is only one typical male pattern of response, while there are three typical female responses that differ as to the occurrence of orgasm. The first pattern shows no orgasm, the second a single orgasm, and the third multiple orgasms. The latter is believed to occur in some women because women do not have the lengthy refractory periods that most men are believed to experience. Masters and Johnson's work is not theoretical; rather, it is based on observation of sexual response in the laboratory. It has been suggested that it would now promote investigation into human sexual response if data were collected in the bedroom rather than in the laboratory.

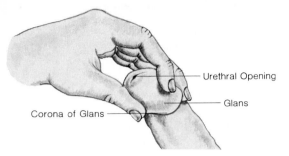

Figure 10.8  To prevent ejaculation, the penis may be gently squeezed as shown. (After Goldstein, *Human Sexuality*, McGraw Hill, 1975.)

## Sexual Dysfunction

There are certain human problems in sexual response that recur often enough to be mentioned here. **Impotency** is the inability to achieve and/or sustain an erection. An impotent man who is unable to participate in sexual intercourse, is not necessarily infertile or sterile for he may be producing sperm that are capable of fertilizing an egg. Impotency can be due to many and diverse reasons but many authorities believe it is often due to psychological causes.[1]

**Premature ejaculation** is defined in various ways, but the definitions imply that a male lacks control over the speed with which he attains orgasm. In other words, barring organic disorders, it is possible for a man to learn to control his excitement by postponing the time when ejaculation becomes inevitable. Men often prefer to delay ejaculation in order to prolong individual sexual experiences for themselves and/or for their partners. It is possible to practice delaying ejaculation and even to have a partner assist in preventing ejaculation. Just before it seems that ejaculation is inevitable, the woman places her thumb and fingers as shown in figure 10.8 and gently applies firm pressure for 3 to 4 seconds or alternately grips the base of the penis and squeezes for several seconds. It is suggested that with time the man will be able to control ejaculation so that it can be delayed.

**Orgasmic dysfunction** occurs when a woman does not experience orgasm. Some authorities suggest that physical causes are rare and that the great majority of cases are interpersonal or psychogenic in origin.[2] However, it has also been suggested by others that if a woman would simply like to increase the frequency of orgasm she might practice contracting the perineal muscles, as described on page 146.[3]

1. E. W. Page et al., *Human Reproduction* (Philadelphia: W. B. Saunders Co., 1976).
2. J. S. DeLora and C. Warren, *Understanding Sexual Interaction* (Boston: Houghton Mifflin, 1977).
3. A. H. Kegel, "Sexual Functions of the Pubococcygeus Muscle," *Western Journal of Surgical and Obstetrical Gynecology 60* (1952): 521.

**Vaginismus** involves involuntary, severe contractions of the muscles surrounding the outer third of the vagina whenever an attempt is made to introduce an object into the vagina. Thus, the vaginal opening remains so tightly closed that intercourse is impossible. It is believed that vaginismus, a rare condition, is due to association of pain or fear with vaginal penetration.[4]

## Fertilization

If intercourse is accompanied by ejaculation, sperm are normally deposited at the rear of the vagina in the region of the cervix (fig. 10.5). The semigelatinous seminal fluid protects the sperm from the acid of the vagina for some minutes, after which they are killed unless they have managed to enter the uterus. Whether or not they enter depends in part on the consistency of the cervical mucus. Three to four days prior to ovulation and on the day of ovulation, the mucus is watery and the sperm can penetrate it easily. During the other days of the cycle, the mucus has a sticky consistency and the sperm can rarely penetrate it.

Fertilization normally occurs in the upper third of the oviduct and a small percentage of sperm (perhaps one hundred thousand) usually arrive there within five to thirty minutes. It is believed that uterine and oviduct contractions transport the sperm and that the prostaglandins within seminal fluid may promote these contractions. Swimming action seems to be important only when the sperm are in the vicinity of the egg.

Since the oocyte is surrounded by a mass of follicular cells and the zona pellucida membrane, it is difficult for a sperm nucleus to gain entrance into the egg cytoplasm. In order to accomplish penetration, the sperm must undergo capacitation by being exposed to the female reproductive tract for several hours. It's been suggested that capacitation involves activation of the enzyme within the sperm acrosome. In any case, the acrosome releases its content of enzyme as the sperm penetrates the outer layers of the egg (fig. 7.3). As soon as a single sperm head has made its way into the region of the cytoplasm, the zona pellucida undergoes a marked and rapid chemical transformation that makes it impossible for other sperm to enter. If by chance other sperm have already entered, then development does not occur. The sperm nucleus moves through the cytoplasm and fuses with the egg nucleus, which has just undergone the second meiotic division. Fertilization is now complete. If fertilization does not occur, the oocyte does not finish meiosis and disintegrates instead.

The fertilized egg, more properly called the zygote, has the diploid number of chromosomes and begins development. The developing zygote travels very slowly down the oviduct to the uterus, where it implants itself in the prepared uterine lining (fig. 10.9). Upon implantation, the female is pregnant.

4. DeLora and Warren, *Understanding Sexual Interaction.*

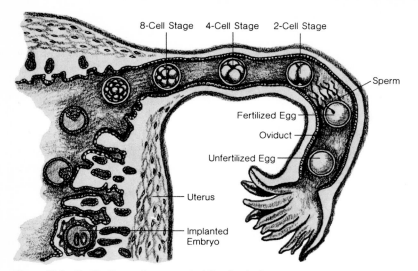

Figure 10.9   Fertilization and movement of the developing
zygote down the oviduct to the uterus where it implants itself.
(After Mader, *Inquiry into Life*, 2d edition.)

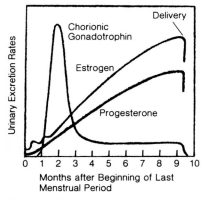

Figure 10.10   Urinary excretion of estrogen, progesterone,
and chorionic gonadotropin during pregnancy. Urinary excretion
rates are an indication of blood concentrations of these
hormones.

If pregnancy does occur, the uterine lining is maintained and menstruation does not normally occur. Menstruation ceases because the outer layer of cells around the embryo produces the gonadotropic hormone HCGTH, which prevents the normal degeneration of the corpus luteum and instead stimulates it to secrete even larger quantities of progesterone.

The corpus luteum is maintained for about three to six months until the placenta is fully developed. The placenta (fig. 10.10) originates from both maternal and fetal tissue and is the region where there is an exchange of molecules between fetal and maternal blood, although there is rarely a mixing of the two types of blood. The umbilical cord stretches between the fetus and the placenta and contains blood vessels that carry oxygen and nutrients to the fetus and carbon dioxide and nitrogen waste to the placenta.

After its formation, the placenta continues production of human chorionic gonadotrophic hormone (HCGTH) and begins production of progesterone and estrogen (fig. 10.10). The latter hormones have two effects—they shut down the anterior pituitary so that no new follicles are started and they maintain the lining of the uterus so that the corpus luteum is no longer needed.

Pregnancy Tests

Pregnancy tests, which are readily available in hospitals, clinics, and now even drug and grocery stores, are based on the fact that HCGTH is present in the blood and urine of a pregnant woman. Pregnancy tests that utilize a blood sample will give a positive result a few days earlier than the urine test, which is not usually performed until two weeks after a missed menstrual period.

*Blood Tests*   A blood sample is allowed to coagulate and the serum that remains is used for the test. Radioactive HCGTH is added and allowed to compete with serum HCGTH for binding with corpus luteum cells or with HCGTH antibodies, depending on the particular test. The amount of bound radioactive HCGTH as opposed to nonradioactive HCGTH from the serum determines if the woman is pregnant.

*Urine Test.*   The most common pregnancy test in use today requires a urine specimen. *HCGTH antibodies* are added to the urine and they either react with the HCGTH in the specimen or with particles coated with HCGTH which are also added. If the particles do react with the HCGTH antibodies, clumping occurs. This clumping indicates that the woman is not pregnant.

The physical signs that might prompt a woman to have a pregnancy test are cessation of menstruation, increase in frequency of urination, morning sickness, and increase in the size and fullness of the breasts, as well as the development of a dark coloration of the areolae.

## Summary

The penis has three longitudinal masses of erectile tissue that fill with blood when the male is sexually aroused. Erection is controlled by sexual response centers in the spinal cord and brain. The expulsion phase of ejaculation occurs when rhythmical contractions of the ischiocavernosus and bulbocavernosus muscles forcibly expell semen from the penis.

In the female, the clitoris and labia minora also contain erectile tissue and the perineal muscles (bulbocavernosus and levator ani muscles) contract rhythmically during sexual excitement.

Vasocongestion and myotonia are thus seen to be important parts of orgasm, which actually includes reactions of the entire body. Masters and Johnson have identified and described four phases of sexual response— excitement, plateau, orgasmic, and resolution. They believe that females are more apt than males to have multiple orgasms.

Sperm can penetrate cervical mucus at the time of ovulation. During their passage through the female reproductive tract the sperm undergo capacitation so that when the sperm contact the egg the acrosomes release an enzyme that allows them to penetrate the zona pellucida. Only one sperm head actually enters the egg and this sperm nucleus fuses with the egg nucleus, which has just undergone the second meiotic division. The zygote begins to develop into an embryo, which travels down the oviduct to imbed itself in the uterine lining. Cells surrounding the embryo produce HCGTH and the presence of this hormone indicates that the female is pregnant.

## Terms

corpora cavernosa

corpus spongiosum

ejaculation

emission

erection

expulsion

fertilization

HCGTH

impotency

myotonia

orgasm

perineum

placenta

vaginismus

vasocongestion

## Review

1. Name four different positions for sexual intercourse and discuss advantages and disadvantages for each.
2. Describe the anatomy and physiology of the male and female perineum.
3. Discuss the physical processes of erection and ejaculation.
4. What two physiological states are observed as accompanying or preceding orgasm? Give an example of each in the male and female.
5. Masters and Johnson have listed four phases of sexual response, name them. What events have been associated with each phase?
6. How do Masters and Johnson diagram the male sexual response? The female sexual response? Compare and contrast these patterns.
7. Describe the process of fertilization and the events immediately following.
8. Explain the absence of menstruation during pregnancy.
9. What are the most commonly used pregnancy tests today?

# 11 Development and Birth

The nine months required for human development are commonly divided into two portions: embryonic development and fetal development. During **embryonic development**, the embryo acquires organ systems and during **fetal development**, there is a refinement of these systems. One of the first events in human development is the establishment of two *extraembryonic membranes*, the amnion and the chorion (fig. 11.1).

Extraembryonic Membranes

The developing human being is enveloped by two tissue layers called **extraembryonic membranes** because they will not be a part of the baby at birth. The inner of the two membranes, the **amnion**, provides a fluid environment for the developing embryo and fetus. It is a remarkable fact that all animals, even land-dwelling humans, develop in water. Amniocentesis (p. 16) is the process by

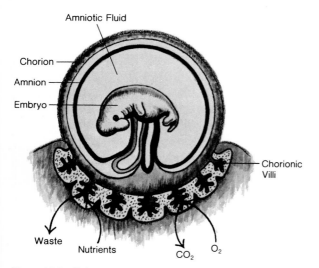

Figure 11.1 Embryo surrounded by two extraembryonic membranes: the amnion and chorion. (After Mader, *Inquiry into Life*, 2d edition.)

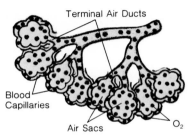

Figure 11.2   After birth, oxygen (circles) moves from the air
sacs of the lungs into the blood. (After Mader, *Inquiry into Life,*
2d edition.)

which amniotic fluid, and the fetal cells floating therein, are withdrawn so that
the chromosomes and biochemical properties of the fluid and cells may be
examined for possible inherited defects. One authority describes the functions
of amniotic fluid in this way:

The colorless amniotic fluid by which the fetus is surrounded serves many
purposes. It prevents the walls of the uterus from cramping the fetus and
allows it unhampered growth and movement. It encompasses the fetus with a
fluid of constant temperature which is a marvelous insulator against cold and
heat. Above all, it acts as an excellent shock absorber. A blow on the
mother's abdomen merely jolts the fetus, and it floats away.[1]

The fetus, immersed in amniotic fluid, cannot breathe air, and the lungs,
which function in adult life to bring oxygen to the blood and take carbon dioxide
away from the blood (fig. 11.2), do not function in the fetus. Instead, oxygen
is absorbed by the fetal blood and carbon dioxide is given off by fetal blood
at the outer extraembryonic membrane, the **chorion.**

In addition to oxygen, the fetus requires a supply of nutrient molecules (for
example, sugar and amino acids). After birth, humans acquire nutrients by eating
food, which is digested to small molecules or chemicals that enter the bloodstream at the small intestines (fig. 11.3). The fetus does not eat food; instead,
nutrient molecules cross the chorion where they enter the fetal blood. Since the
fetus does not digest food, defecation is not necessary, but nitrogenous metabolic wastes such as urea must exit from fetal blood. While this function is
taken care of by the kidneys in the adult (fig. 11.4), in the fetus nitrogenous
wastes exit at the chorion.

1. A. F. Guttmacher, *Pregnancy, Birth and Family Planning*
   (New York: New American Library, 1974), p. 74.

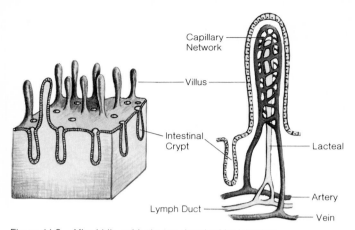

Capillary Network

Villus

Intestinal Crypt

Lacteal

Lymph Duct

Artery

Vein

Figure 11.3  After birth, nutrients are absorbed by intestinal villi (fingerlike projections of the intestinal wall) into the blood. (After Volpe, *Man, Nature, and Society,* 2d edition.)

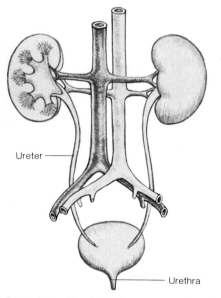

Ureter

Urethra

Figure 11.4  After birth, nitrogenous waste molecules leave the blood and enter kidney tubules to be excreted by way of the urinary tract. (After Mader, *Inquiry into Life,* 2d edition.)

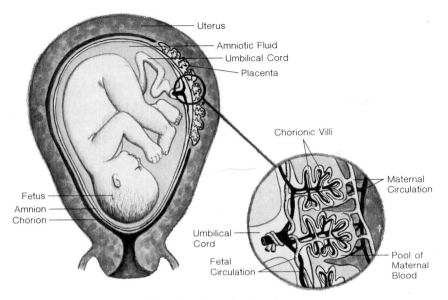

Figure 11.5 At the placenta, fetal circulation and maternal circulation lie in close proximity so that waste molecules pass from the fetal to the maternal circulation and nutrient molecules pass in the opposite direction. (After Mader, *Inquiry into Life*, 2d edition.)

## Placenta

The chorion is in intimate contact with maternal tissue because the developing embryo implanted itself in the uterine wall. On one side of the chorion there is mother's blood and on the other side there is embryonic blood (fig. 11.1) Oxygen and nutrient molecules pass from mother's blood to baby's blood while carbon dioxide and waste molecules pass from baby's blood to mother's blood. The term **placenta** is used to refer to the region where this exchange takes place. The placenta has two portions: the embryonic and later fetal half is chorionic tissue and the maternal half is uterine tissue (fig. 11.5).

While it is obvious that there is no nervous connection between the pregnant woman and her child (thus, fear experienced by a pregnant woman cannot affect the child), it is also apparent that chemicals present in woman's blood can pass to fetal blood. Medications and other drugs present in expectant mother's blood do pass to baby's blood. The most notorious example of the harmful developmental effects due to this are the thalidomide babies (fig. 11.6). An estimated 10,000 children were born with deformed arms and sometimes legs because their mothers had taken this sedative during their pregnancy.

We also know that drug addicts and alcoholics have babies who display withdrawal symptoms and that smokers have underweight babies. Therefore, it seems reasonable to suggest that a pregnant woman should be very careful

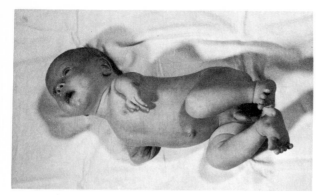

Figure 11.6  Thalidomide baby. (Source: Professor W. Lenz, editor of *Archives of Environmental Health*.)

about taking drugs of any sort because of the effect they may have on her developing child. Also, the pregnant woman should avoid X-ray therapy. Dividing cells are particularly susceptible to damage by x ray and, as we shall see, cell division is absolutely essential to development.

In addition to drugs, disease organisms can pass from the expectant mother's blood to her baby's blood. For example, an embryo can contract syphilis from its mother (p. 200). Rubella (German measles) is also an early deformer of embryonic development. Any woman who has not been previously immunized and contracts rubella during the first three months of her pregnancy may wish to consider an abortion because the virus may cause congenital malformations.

Drugs and disease often affect embyonic rather than fetal development because this is the period of time when structures are first appearing. Unfortunately, this is also the time when women are most likely not to realize that they are pregnant. Therefore, especially when birth control is not being practiced, the prospective mother should carefully watch her health and intake of drugs.

Umbilical Cord

While it may seem that the **umbilical cord** (fig. 11.6) travels from the intestines to the placenta, actually the umbilical cord is simply taking fetal blood to and from the placenta. The umbilical cord is the lifeline of the fetus because it contains the umbilical arteries and vein, which transport waste molecules (carbon dioxide and urea) to the placenta for disposal and take oxygen and nutrient molecules from the placenta to the rest of the fetal circulatory system (fig. 11.7).

Fetal circulation contains other features not seen in adult circulation. In the adult, for example, blood entering the right side of the heart passes to the lungs for oxygenation before returning to the left side of the heart. In the fetus, blood

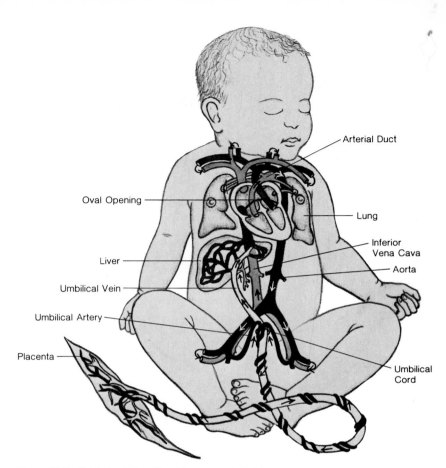

Figure 11.7 Fetal circulation. Blood is oxygenated at the placenta and enters the umbilical vein, which joins with the vena cava. From the vena cava, blood enters the right side of the heart and passes directly to the left side by way of the oval window or else enters the pulmonary trunk and passes to the aorta by way of the arterial duct. In either case, blood does not go to the lungs. (After Mader, *Inquiry into Life,* 2d edition.)

moves directly from the right side of the heart to the left side of the heart by way of an opening called the oval opening. Any blood that does happen to leave the right side of the heart still bypasses the lungs by entering a connector vessel called the arterial duct.

**Development**, which starts with a single cell, proceeds from the simple to the complex. First, the single cell becomes a number of cells by the process of mitosis; then these cells differentiate into tissues and finally the tissues become

## Chart 11.1

Human Development

| Time | Events |
|------|--------|
| *Embryonic Development* | |
| First week | Fertilization. Cell division begins and continues. First membrane appears. |
| Second week | Implantation. Second membrane appears. Embryo has tissues. Placenta begins. |
| Third week | Nervous system begins. Yolk sac and blood vessels are present. Placenta is well formed. |
| Fourth week | Limb buds begin. Heart is noticeable and beating. Nervous system is prominent. Embryo has tail. Other systems begin. |
| Fifth week | 1/12″. Embryo is curved. Head is large. Limb buds show divisions. Nose, eyes, and ears are noticeable. |
| Sixth week. | 1/4″. Fingers and toes are present. Cartilaginous skeleton. |
| Two months | 1/2″. All systems are developing. Bone is replacing cartilage. Refinement of facial features. |
| *Fetal Development* | |
| Third month | 3″ (1 ounce). Possible to distinguish sex. Fingernails. |
| Fourth month | 8.5″ (6 ounces). Skeleton visible. Hair begins to appear. |
| Fifth month | 12″ (1 lb.). Mother can feel movement. Protective cheesy coating begins to be deposited. Heartbeat can be heard. |
| Sixth month | 14″ (2 lbs.). Body is covered with fine hair. Skin is wrinkled and red. |
| Seventh month | 16″ (4 lbs.). Testes descend into scrotum. Eyes are open. |
| Eighth month | Body hair begins to disappear. Subcutaneous fat begins to be deposited. |
| Ninth month | 20″ (7 lbs.). Ready for birth. |

organized into organs. Development is an orderly process by which each preceding event seems to trigger the event that follows. Step-by-step, the zygote becomes a complex newborn (chart 11.1). Embryonic development is the term used for development from conception to the end of the second month and fetal development refers to the final seven months.

Embryonic Development

*First Week*

Immediately after fertilization, the zygote divides repeatedly. The resulting cells arrange themselves so that there is an inner cell mass surrounded by a layer of cells that will become the chorion (fig. 11.8a). The early appearance of the chorion emphasizes the complete dependence of the developing embryo on this membrane. The inner cell mass will become the baby.

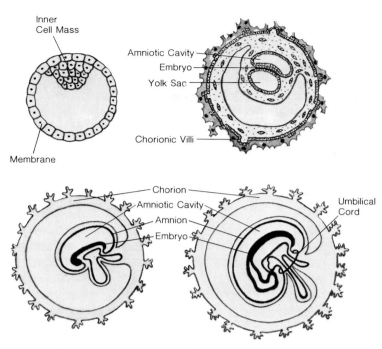

Figure 11.8  Stages in the development of human embryo showing early appearance of chorion and amnion (top); and development of the umbilical cord (bottom).

As cell division takes place, the embryo passes down the oviduct to the uterus where it embeds itself at about the seventh day (fig. 10.10). With implantation, pregnancy has now taken place, and the placenta begins formation.

*Second week*
The ever-growing number of cells are now arranged in tissues and the amniotic cavity is seen above the embryo. Two vestigial extraembryonic membranes, the **yolk sac** and **allantois**, make their appearance briefly but later become a part of the umbilical cord that is now forming (fig. 11.8).

*Third week*
Organs are already developing, including the nerve cord and heart. The nervous system and circulatory system have begun.

*One month*
The woman's menstrual flow is two weeks late and the placenta has begun producing **h**uman **c**horionic **g**onadotropic **h**ormone (HCGTH), which maintains

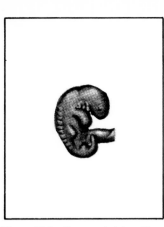

Figure 11.9  Four-week fetus. (Source for figures 11.9–11.14:
Original artwork courtesy Carnation Company, Los Angeles,
California. © Carnation Co., 1962.)

the corpus luteum and the uterine lining. The fetal half of the placenta, the chorion, has treelike villi that project into the uterine tissue. As the fetus develops, these villi enlarge at one location only, although they may eventually take up as much as 50 percent of the uterus (fig. 11.5).

The embryo has a nonhuman appearance largely due to the presence of a tail but also because the arms and legs, which begin as limb buds, resemble paddles. The head is much larger than the rest of the embryo and the whole embryo bends under its weight (fig. 11.9). Eyes, ears, and nose are just appearing. The enlarged heart beats and the bulging liver produces red blood cells for the formation of blood that will carry nutrients to the developing organs and wastes from the developing organs.

### Two Months
At the end of two months, the tail has disappeared and the arms and legs are better formed with fingers and toes apparent (fig. 11.10). The head is very large; the nose is flat; the eyes are far apart; and the ears are distinctively present. Internally, all major organs have appeared. Embryonic development is now finished.

### Fetal Development
Fetal development represents simply a refinement of embryonic development (figs. 11.11–11.14), and we cannot escape the fact that at the end of embryonic development a living, functioning human is present in the uterus. The woman's period is only six weeks late and already her developing baby has all of its major organs!

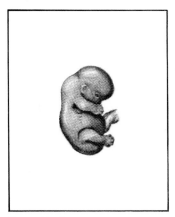

Figure 11.10    Eight-week fetus.

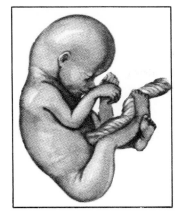

Figure 11.11    Three-to-four-month fetus.

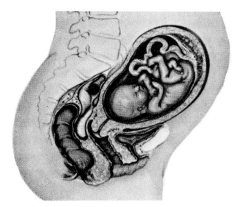

Figure 11.12    Four-to-five-month fetus.

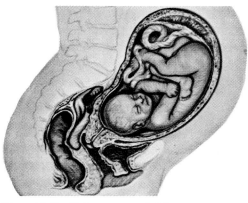

Figure 11.13    Six-to-seven-month fetus.

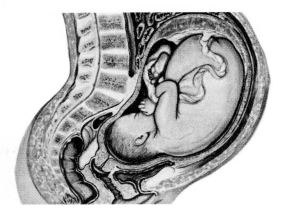

Figure 11.14   Eight-to-nine-month fetus.

Chart 11.1 gives the main events of fetal development. Of major interest may be the fact that during the third month it would be possible to tell the sex of the fetus by visual examination. During the fourth month, the baby is covered by a fine, downlike hair and a bony skeleton has appeared. During the fifth month, the expectant mother can feel the movements of the fetus and the doctor can hear the heartbeat. During the six month, the baby is covered by a heavy protective cheesy coating called the **vernix caseosa**. By the seventh month very little further development is needed; premature babies at this stage have a fair chance of survival in nurseries staffed by skilled physicians and nurses. Therefore, the baby is said to be viable. During the eighth and ninth months, the baby puts on weight and prepares for its entrance into the world.

## Birth

The uterus characteristically contracts throughout pregnancy. At first, light, often indiscernible contractions last about 20–30 seconds and occur every 15 or 20 minutes, but near the end of pregnancy they become stronger and more frequent so that the woman may falsely think that she is in labor. The onset of true labor is marked by uterine contractions that occur regularly every 15 to 20 minutes and last for 40 seconds or more. **Parturition**, which includes labor and expulsion of the fetus, is usually considered to have three stages. During the **first stage**, the cervix dilates; during the **second**, the baby is born; and during the **third**, the afterbirth is expelled.

The events that cause parturition to begin have been investigated for some time, but there are now new findings. It is believed that the fetal hypothalamus directs the fetal pituitary to produce ACTH (adrenocorticotropin), which in turn stimulates the adrenal gland of the fetus to secrete the hormone cortisone. This hormone brings about the production of prostaglandins in the placenta. Prostaglandins are hormones that have a host of effects on the human body, including contraction of the uterus. It may be too that prostaglandins bring about the release of oxytocin from the maternal pituitary gland. Since oxytocin can cause uterine contractions, either prostaglandins or oxytocin may be given to induce parturition.

Stage I

Prior to this stage or concomitant with it, there may be a "bloody show" caused by the expulsion of a mucus plug from the cervical canal. This plug prevented bacteria and sperm from entering the uterus during the pregnancy.

Uterine contractions during the first stage of labor occur in such a way that the cervical canal slowly disappears (fig. 11.15) as the lower part of the uterus is pulled upward toward the baby's head. This process is called effacement, or "taking up the cervix." With further contractions, the baby's head acts as a wedge to assist cervical dilation. The baby's head usually has a diameter of about 4 inches and therefore the cervix has to dilate to this diameter in order to allow the head to pass through. If it has not occurred already, the amniotic membrane is apt to rupture now, releasing the amniotic fluid, which escapes out the vagina. The first stage of labor ends once the cervix is completely dilated.

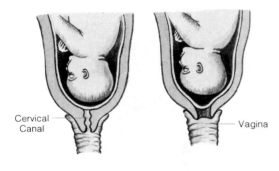

Cervical
Canal                                                      Vagina

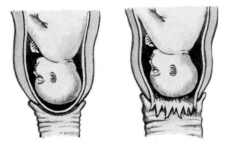

Figure 11.15    Stage I of parturition: effacement.

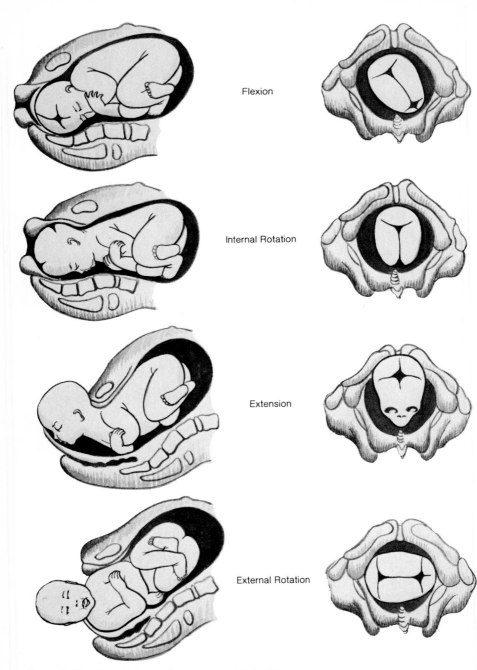

**Flexion**

**Internal Rotation**

**Extension**

**External Rotation**

Figure 11.16   Stage II of parturition: process of birth. (Source: Gordon Bourne and David N. Danforth, *Pregnancy*. Copyright © 1974 by Cassall Ltd.)

## Stage II

During the second stage, the uterine contractions occur every 1–2 minutes and last about 1 minute each. They are accompanied by a desire to push or bear down. As the baby's head gradually descends into the vagina, the desire to push becomes greater. When the baby's head reaches the perineum, it turns so that the back of the head is uppermost (fig. 11.16). Since the vagina may not expand enough to allow passage of the head without tearing, an **episiotomy** is often performed. This incision of the perineum is stitched later and will heal more perfectly than a tear would. The baby's head emerges from the vagina in degrees—first the forehead, then the nose, and finally the mouth and chin, with the neck situated the entire time just behind the front bone of the pelvic girdle (fig. 11.16). As soon as the head is delivered, the baby's shoulders rotate so that the baby looks either to the right or left. The physician may at this time hold the head and guide it downward while one shoulder and then the other emerges. The rest of the baby follows easily.

The baby's first breath accompanies the events that convert fetal circulation to adult circulation. The change in environmental pressure following birth causes blood to circulate to the lungs rather than entering the arterial duct. The arterial duct contracts and never relaxes. Blood returning from the lungs to the heart exerts pressure against a flap that permanently closes off the oval window. If these circulatory changes do not occur or if there is some other cardiac defect, surgery may be required.

Once the baby is breathing normally, the umbilical cord is cut and tied, severing the child from the placenta. The stump of the cord shrivels and leaves a scar, which is the navel.

## Stage III

The placenta, or afterbirth, is delivered during the third stage of labor (fig. 11.17). About 15 minutes after delivery of the baby, uterine muscular contractions shrink the uterus and dislodge the placenta. The placenta is then expelled into the vagina. As soon as the placenta and its membranes are delivered, the third stage of labor is complete.

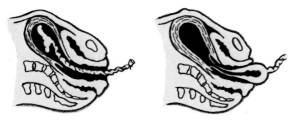

Figure 11.17    Stage III of parturition: delivery of afterbirth.

*Prepared childbirth.*

Some doctors and expectant couples feel that nervous system depressants may be harmful not only to the expectant mother but to the baby as well. This sentiment, together with a desire to enjoy and share the process of giving birth, has given impetus to the prepared childbirth movement. Usually couples who wish to practice prepared childbirth using the methods espoused by Dr. Fernand Lamaze and others attend several teaching sessions in which they learn about the events of labor and delivery, the phenomenon of conditioned pain, and suggestions for behavior during labor and delivery.

It is believed that the woman may help prevent discomfort during labor by concentrating on mild, shallow breathing at the time of contractions. This breathing method prevents the diaphragm from exerting pressure on the abdominal organs and guarantees an adequate supply of oxygen for uterine contraction. When delivery begins and the woman feels a great need to push, her partner coaches her to use deep inhalation along with a controlled type of pushing at the time of each strong contraction. Advocates of the Lamaze method of prepared childbirth feel that this active participation on the part of the couple will not only help the woman overlook discomfort but will also give the pair the pleasant reward of seeing the baby when it first appears.

## Reproduction in the Laboratory

Intercourse with ejaculation need not precede fertilization, development, and birth. Artificial insemination in which sperm are introduced into the vagina by means of a cannula (tube) has been practiced for many years. Each year an estimated 25,000 American women receive sperm from anonymous donors whose pedigrees have been carefully checked for hereditary defects, and about 10,000 children are born because of subsequent conceptions.

Eggs can also be fertilized in laboratory glassware during a process called *in vitro* fertilization. To obtain the required oocytes, the woman is given a dose of HCGTH, which will cause multiple ovulations in nonpregnant women. Then, abdominal surgery is performed to acquire the preovulatory oocytes, which look like bulges on the surface of the ovary. To see the ovaries, a small incision allows the insertion of a laparascope, which is much like a small telescope with a cold light source, and the oocytes can subsequently be removed by a suction tube introduced through a second incision.

Sperm from a male donor are placed in a salt solution where they undergo capacitation. When the oocytes are introduced, fertilization occurs. The resultant embryos are transferred to a different solution and are kept in an atmosphere of low oxygen tension. Sometime between two and four days after fertilization, the developing embryo may be inserted into the uterus of a woman who is in the secretory phase of her menstrual cycle. Hopefully, it will implant itself and develop normally. Louise Brown, born July 25, 1978 in Oldham, England, is the first-known baby ever to be conceived in laboratory glassware.

Some lay persons and scientists do not approve of *in vitro* fertilization because they do not believe that investigators should control human life. Other lay persons and scientists believe that increased control over human life will be of benefit to mankind. Currently, *in vitro* fertilization would be most helpful to couples troubled with infertility due to blockage of the woman's oviducts.

Birth of a baby following *in vitro* fertilization is not the same as cloning. **Cloning** has come to mean the production of an offspring with exactly the same chromosome makeup as another normally sexually reproducing organism. This procedure has been accomplished in frogs. The nucleus of a frog's egg is destroyed by ultraviolet radiation and the nucleus from a tadpole cell is inserted into the egg. The diploid egg begins to divide and a tadpole results that is just like the one from which the nucleus was taken. It has been *speculated* that cloning might be possible in human beings. A nucleus, taken from a cell of the individual to be cloned, would be placed in a nucleus-free egg. Embryonic development would follow and the embryo could then be introduced into the uterus of a volunteer where it would finish development, or the embryo could develop in an artificial womb. Artificial wombs, much like incubators filled with synthetic amniotic fluid, have been developed and animal fetuses have been kept alive for several days within such a womb. Regardless of where development occurs, the newborn baby would have the same genetic potential as the donor of the diploid nucleus.

There has been much speculation about the possibility of cloning well-known personalities so that there could be many copies of world-famous persons. However, the possibility of cloning adults is still remote because an adult cell nucleus is not likely to function in the same manner as an embryonic nucleus, when placed in an enucleated egg. Nuclei taken from specialized adult cells contain genes that were turned off as specialization took place. These genes would have to be stimulated to function again, if cloning of adults were to become a reality. Most scientists feel that cloning is still an unlikely procedure for many years to come.

Genetic Engineering

In contrast to reproductive experiments, genetic engineering refers to (1) the correction of gene defects and (2) the manipulation of genes to control human evolution. On occasion, it has been possible to treat genetic defects prenatally so that a healthy baby has been born rather than a defective one. For example, if amniocentesis shows that a baby is incapable of making a particular metabolite, the mother can supply this substance to the child by way of the placenta if she takes massive doses. This is a form of genetic engineering, but more dramatic procedures have been proposed. Recombinant DNA research has permitted the introduction of man-made genes into bacteria where they function normally (p. 76). Therefore, it has been suggested that normal genes needed to correct a genetic defect could be introduced into the sperm and egg just before, or into the zygote, just after *in vitro* fertilization. It has even been speculated that it might eventually be possible to develop human genes that would code for desired traits, such as more intelligence, and that these could be introduced into developing zygotes in order to influence the course of human evolution. Such a possibility is still remote. The one thing that can presently be done to try to control human evolution is for everyone to try to bring into the world humans who are as genetically and physically fit as possible and who will receive the care that each human deserves.

---

## Summary

Human development consists of embryonic and fetal development. During the first two months of pregnancy, the extraembryonic membranes appear and serve important functions and the embryo acquires organ systems. During the remaining months, the time of fetal development, there is a refinement of these systems (chart 11.1).

The fetus, which lies within the amnion surrounded by fluid, is connected to the placenta by means of the umbilical cord. Partuition, or birth, has three phases. During the first stage, the cervix dilates to allow passage of the baby's head and body. The amnion usually bursts sometime during this stage. During the second stage, the baby is born and the umbilical cord is cut. As the baby takes its first breath, anatomical changes convert fetal circulation to adult circulation. During the third stage, the placenta is delivered.

Because of scientific advances, it is possible to artifically assist the process of fertilization and development. Artificial insemination is a common practice, but recently fertilization has been carried out *in vitro*. Birth of a baby following *in vitro* fertilization is not cloning, which is the production of an offspring with the same chromosomal makeup of another human. Genetic engineering includes correction of gene defects and manipulation of genes to control human evolution. Prenatal correction of gene defects has been attempted, but the possibity of gene manipulation to control evolution is remote.

## Terms

| | |
|---|---|
| afterbirth | extraembryonic membranes |
| amnion | fetus |
| arterial duct | labor |
| chorion | oval opening |
| cloning | partuition |
| effacement | umbilical cord |
| embryo | |

## Review

1. Name the two extraembryonic membranes and give a function for each.
2. Name three organs that do not function in the fetus and describe how their functions are accomplished by the placenta.
3. What time during pregnancy does a woman have to be the most careful about the intake of medications and other drugs?
4. Describe the structure and function of the umbilical cord.
5. Specifically, what events normally occur during the first, second, third, and fourth weeks of development? What events normally happen during the second through the ninth months?
6. In general, describe the events of embryonic and fetal development.
7. What are the three stages of birth? Describe the happenings during each stage.

# 12

# Birth Control and Infertility

The use of birth control (contraceptive) methods decreases the probability of pregnancy. One authority estimates that the normal, healthy young woman in her early twenties who is having unprotected intercourse three or more times per week with a normal, healthy man has a chance of becoming pregnant according to the following schedule.

30% will be pregnant within *one month*
45% will be pregnant within *two months*
55% will be pregnant within *three months*
65% will be pregnant within *six months*
80% will be pregnant within *one year*
85% will be pregnant within *two years or longer*[1]

A common way to discuss pregnancy rate is to indicate the number of pregnancies expected per 100 (or 1,000) women per year. According to the above statistics, we could expect 80 young women out of 100 women who are regularly engaging in unprotected intercourse to be pregnant within a year. Another way to discuss birth control methods is to indicate their effectiveness (fig. 12.1), in which case the emphasis is placed on the number of women who would not get pregnant. For example, with the least effective method given in figure 12.1 we would expect that 70 women out of 100 would not get pregnant, while 30 women would get pregnant within a year.

## Group I

Sterilization

**Sterilization** as a means of birth control is a surgical procedure that renders the individual incapable of reproduction. The operations do not affect the secondary sex characteristics of the individual, nor do they necessarily affect the

1. G. Bourne and D. Danforth, *Pregnancy* (New York: Harper & Row, Publishers, 1972), p. 523.

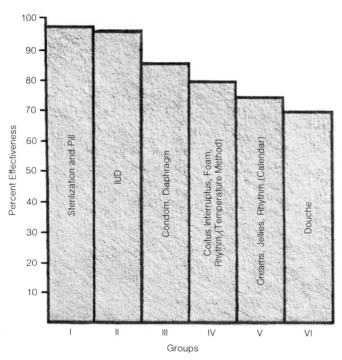

Figure 12.1 Effectiveness of birth control procedures and devices. (Data based on Guttmacher, Alan F. *Pregnancy, Birth, and Family Planning,* New York, New American Library, 1973.)

sex performance. Successful vasectomy in the male and tubal ligation in the female allow the individual to engage in sexual activities with absolutely no fear of pregnancy.

*Vasectomy.*

As the name implies, a vasectomy consists of cutting the vas (ductus) deferentia (fig. 12.2). The operation is very simple. Two small incisions (sometimes one incision) are made on the scrotum to expose the spermatic cords. The vas deferentia are carefully separated from the other structures in the spermatic cords and a small section of each is removed. Each end is then sealed so that sperm will be unable to travel to the urethra.

Vasectomies performed on well-adjusted and healthy individuals do not generally alter sexual motivation, ability to maintain an erection, or ejaculation of semen. However, there has been some concern about an unexpected reaction: antibodies against a man's own sperm have been found in the blood following

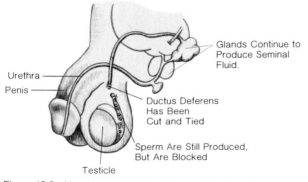

Urethra

Penis

Glands Continue to
Produce Seminal
Fluid.

Ductus Deferens
Has Been
Cut and Tied

Sperm Are Still Produced,
But Are Blocked

Testicle

Figure 12.2   Vasectomy involves cutting and blocking the
ductus deferentia, formerly called the vas deferentia.

vasectomy. It has been hypothesized that due to the build-up of sperm in the epididymides, sperm are engulfed by white cells that later enter the bloodstream. If remnants of the sperm enter the blood from the white cells, then antibodies are formed against them. These antibodies will thereafter invade the testes to attack sperm.

Vasectomy should be considered an irreversible operation because (1) resectioning the sperm ducts may be difficult and (2) fertility is usually reduced, perhaps due to the antibody reaction mentioned above.

*Tubal ligation.*

In this operative procedure, the oviducts are cut and/or sealed (fig. 12.3), thereby preventing sperm from reaching the egg, which must halt on the far side of the obstruction. **Tubal ligation** can be accomplished by abdominal surgery, but less traumatic methods have been developed in recent years.

**Laparascopy** requires only two small incisions that can be covered with adhesive bandages. First, a local anesthetic is given and the abdomen is distended with an inert gas in order to give the physician a clear view of the oviducts. A small incision is made near the navel and the laparascope (like a small telescope with a "cold" light source) is introduced through this cut. Further down, a tiny surgical knife inserted through a second incision is used to cut and remove a small portion of each tube.

An even-newer method is called **hysteroscopic** sterilization. In this procedure, a telescopic device is inserted into the uterus (hystera means womb) by way of the vagina. This time the oviducts are sealed with an electric current where they enter the uterus. If the operation is successful, scar tissue forms and blocks the tubes. The failure rate, which has been as high as 25 percent, is reduced if the operation is performed early in the woman's menstrual cycle before the uterine lining has had time to thicken.

Human Reproduction

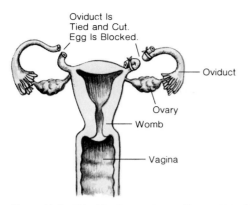

Figure 12.3   Tubal ligation involves cutting and blocking the oviducts.

Like vasectomy, tubal ligation should be considered an irreversible operation. It's possible to resection the tubes, but this requires abdominal surgery and the resultant fertility is not high.

The Pill

The **birth control pill** is usually a combination of estrogen and progesterone that is taken for twenty-one days out of a twenty-eight day cycle. Either no pill or an inactive pill is taken for seven days. The estrogen and progesterone in the pill effectively shut down the pituitary production of both FSH and LH by the feedback mechanism. Theoretically, since the pituitary is not producing FSH, no follicle begins to develop in the ovary, ovulation does not occur, and pregnancy cannot occur. Without the maturation of a follicle, the ovaries do not produce the female sex hormone, but the pill provides these hormones for the patient.

Aside from this primary action of the pill, there are *three secondary actions* that would most likely prevent pregnancy should ovulation happen to occur. The pill prevents the cervical mucus from entering its midcycle thin, watery phase. Instead, the mucus remains sticky and fairly impenetrable by sperm. The hormones in the pill might affect the transport of an embryo down the oviducts so that it would not arrive in the uterus at the proper time for implantation. The pill also prevents normal build-up of the lining of the uterus and therefore an embryo would be unable to implant itself. This action of the pill accounts for the fact that the menses lasts fewer days and the flow is lighter when a woman takes the pill.

Since the pill has one primary action and three secondary actions to prevent pregnancy, it is highly effective. It has been calculated that there should be no more than 1 pregnancy per 1,000 women using the pill. However, the pregnancy rate is actually 5–7 pregnancies per 1,000 because women do not always carefully follow the directions for use.

## Side Effects

Both beneficial and adverse side effects have been linked to the pill. Women report relief of discomforts associated with the menses and also relief of acne. They also report several minor adverse side affects that are not generally considered to be injurious to health. Many of these are similar to symptoms associated with early pregnancy and are therefore thought to be related to the estrogen in the pill. They include nausea, vomiting, painful breast swelling, and irregular spotting or bleeding. Less common complaints are weight gain, headache, dizziness, and sometimes *chloasma*, areas of darkened skin on the face, particularly over the cheekbones. Most often these side effects, except for chloasma, either diminish or disappear by the second or third pill cycle.

A well-documented *serious side effect* and therefore a major side effect of the pill is an increased incidence of blood clotting within the vessels. Blood clotting normally occurs only when a vessel has been cut, but it can abnormally occur within an intact vessel. If the clot remains stationary and obstructs the flow of blood where formed, it is called a **thrombus**. If the clot is carried to a smaller vessel where it prevents flow, it is called an **embolus**. If the clogged vessel serves a vital organ such as the lung, brain, or heart, serious illness or death may result.

*Thromboembolism* in women on the pill has been studied extensively in England and the United States. These studies compare the incidence of thromboembolism in two groups of women—one group is taking the pill and the other group is not taking the pill. The number of women who are hospitalized or who die due to thromboembolism is about 5–7 times greater in the group taking the pill than in the group not taking the pill. The higher increased incidence occurs when the group of women taking the pill are thirty-five to forty years of age and/or are smokers. If the group of women both smoke and have some other risk factor such as hypertension the chance of thromboembolism jumps to 78 times as great for a pill user as for a nonuser. It is therefore recommended that these women consider another form of contraception.

People who are against birth control often use these studies to suggest that all women should not take the pill. Proponents of oral contraception compare the risk with that of pregnancy and illegal abortions in order to suggest that oral contraception is safer than pregnancy and illegal abortions.

There has been no evidence of a higher incidence of *cancer* in women taking the pill. When estrogen is given in high continuous doses to strains of animals that are prone to breast cancer, there is an increased incidence of this type of cancer in these animals. Therefore, some investigators believe that there will be an increased incidence of cancer in women, especially those who have taken the pill for twenty years or so. As yet, there have been no data to support this contention, but it is suggested that women who have had cancer should not take the pill.

Since there are contraindications to taking the pill, it should always be prescribed by a physican only after a careful physical examination; and since there are side effects, it should be taken only under a physician's continuous care.

## Group II

Intrauterine Devices (IUD)

**Intrauterine devices** *(IUD)* (fig. 12.4) are small pieces of molded plastic that are inserted into the uterus by a pyhsician. Some IUDs have copper wire around the stem from which copper is emitted continuously and other IUDs release progesterone. The effectiveness of treated IUDs is higher than that of the plain plasitic ones.

IUDs most likely prevent implantation by the embryo, since there is often an inflammatory reaction where the device presses against the endometrium. Some investigators believe that the IUD alters tubal motility so that the embryo arrives in the uterus before it is properly prepared to receive it. A question arises as to whether an IUD and other birth control methods cause an abortion. Some people believe that preventing an embryo from implanting is an abortion, while others believe that an abortion is the removal of an embryo that is already implanted.

Side Effects

The minor side effects of the IUD are expulsion, pain, irregular bleeding, or profuse menses. The device can be expelled from the uterus usually during menses without the woman realizing it. To guard against this, the IUDs have an attached nylon thread that projects into the vagina; the wearer can note the presence of the thread by the insertion of a finger.

 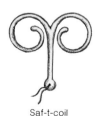 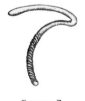

Lippes Loop                    Saf-t-coil                         Copper 7

Figure 12.4   Various types of intrauterine devices.

The major side effects of IUDs are pelvic infection and perforation of the uterus. The infection can usually be treated by suitable antibiotics, but deaths have ocurred. If the device perforates the uterus, it may enter the abdominal cavity. Since an operation would be required to remove it, it is sometimes left undisturbed.

About 3–8 pregnancies a year can be expected per 100 women using the nontreated-type IUD. If pregnancy should occur, it is strongly advised that the device be removed and that an abortion be considered. In 1974 the Department of Health, Education, and Welfare banned the use of the Dalkon Shield, sometimes called the crab, from use in federally supported birth control clinics because of disease related to pregnancy in women who had worn the Dalkon Shield.

## Group III

Diaphragm

The diaphragm (fig. 12.5), or Dutch cap, is a soft rubber or plastic cup with a flexible rim that lodges behind the pubic bone and fits over the cervix. The physician determines the proper diaphragm size; therefore, each woman must be individually fitted. The diaphragm must be inserted into the vagina and properly positioned at most two hours before sexual relations. It must be used with a spermicidal jelly or cream and should be left in place for at least six hours after intercourse.

An allergic reaction to the cap or jelly (cream) is the only known side effect to the use of the diaphragm. There is a higher rate of pregnancy (10–15 pregnancies per 100 women per year) than with the pill or IUD because insertion may require an interruption to lovemaking and the woman does not bother to

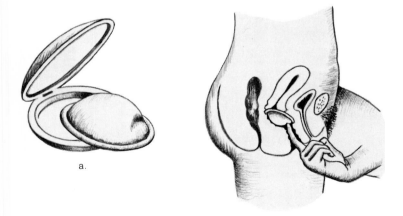

a.

b.

Figure 12.5 Diaphragm. (a) Removal from plastic container; (b) insertion and position after insertion.

Human Reproduction

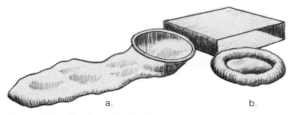

Figure 12.6 Condom. (a) Unrolled and (b) rolled.

use the diaphragm. Some women do not like to handle the genital organs and therefore prefer not to use the diaphragm. However, it is possible to learn to use an inserter to put the diaphragm in place.

Condom

A condom (fig. 12.6) is a thin skin or plastic sheath that fits over the erect penis. The ejaculate is trapped inside the sheath and thus does not enter the vagina. When used in conjunction with a spermicidal foam, cream, or jelly, the protection is better than the condom alone, for which 10–15 unplanned pregnancies a year per 100 women are expected.

There are no side effects to the use of the condom and they may be purchased in a drugstore without a prescription. Condoms are checked during the manufacturing process for any possible defects, therefore, it is believed that their relatively high failure rate is due largely to misuse. The condom must be placed on the penis after it is erect and a small space should be left at the tip to collect the ejaculate. If added lubrication is desired, a nonpetroleum-base jelly, such as a spermicidal jelly or cream, should be used since petroleum products—vaseline, for example—tend to destroy the plastic. Following ejaculation, the upper part of the condom should be held tight against the penis as it is withdrawn from the vagina.

Some men and women feel that the use of the condom not only interrupts the sex act, it also dulls sensations and therefore they prefer one of the other birth control methods. However, the condom is the only means of birth control that offers possible protection against venereal disease, p. 195.

## Groups IV and V

Coitus Interruptus (Withdrawal)

This method of birth control is called **coitus interruptus** because sexual intercourse is abruptly interrupted in order to discharge the semen outside the vagina. Just before orgasm, the male withdraws his penis from the vagina and ejaculates away from the vaginal area. This procedure requires careful timing by the male and he must be sure to direct the penis away from the vagina, as it is possible for sperm deposited near the vagina to work their way in and up the uterus and to the fallopian tubes.

The advantage to coitus interruptus is that it is always available, but the protection is not considered good especially since the first drop of seminal fluid, which is released before orgasm, contains numerous sperm (p. 111). Also, sex relations are unsatisfactory for some because the male has to concentrate on good timing and the sex act is abruptly discontinued. Ten to 20 unplanned pregnancies per 100 women per year are expected with this method of birth control.

## Spermicidal Jellies, Creams, and Foams

These products (fig. 12.7), which contain sperm-killing ingredients, are inserted into the vagina with an applicator up to 30 minutes before intercourse. A fresh application is required for each subsequent intercourse. Used alone, they are not a highly effective means of birth control, but the foam is more effective because it reaches all parts of the vagina, whereas the jellies and creams tend to localize centrally. It is estimated that 15–25 out of 100 women become pregnant each year using this method of birth control.

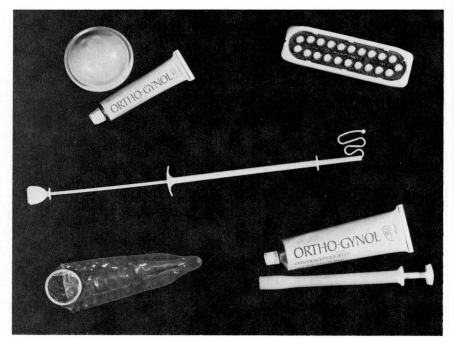

Figure 12.7   Contraceptives.

There are no serious side effects with the use of these products and they are readily available without prescription in the drugstore. Some women are allergic to certain spermicidal agents and must switch to a new product or discontinue using them. Some couples prefer a different method of birth control because of the low protection rate and because insertion might tend to interrupt sexual relations.

Rhythm Method

The rhythm method of birth control is based on the fact that a woman ovulates only once a month (p. 122) and that the egg and sperm are viable for a limited number of hours or days. The day of ovulation can vary from month to month and the fertility of the egg and sperm varies perhaps monthly but certainly from person to person. Therefore, the so-called safe period for intercourse without fear of pregnancy cannot be absolutely determined by the use of a calendar alone. However, the following procedure can be utilized by those who are willing to risk an unexpected pregnancy.

1. Keep a record of the length of the monthly cycle for a year. Note the shortest and the longest cycle.
2. Subtract 18 from the number of days in the shortest cycle. This is the day on which the unsafe period begins.
3. Subtract 11 from the number of days in the longest cycle. This is the day on which the unsafe period ends.

For example, suppose Mary Smith's shortest cycle for the year was 25 days and the longest was 29: 25 − 18 = 7 and 29 − 11 = 18. No intercourse should take place between the seventh and nineteenth days of each cycle (fig. 12.8). Using this method, 15–30 pregnancies per 100 women per year are expected.

A more reliable way to practice the rhythm method of birth control is to await the day of ovulation each month and then wait three more days before engaging in intercourse. The day of ovulation can possibly be determined by one of the following methods:

1. Body temperature is lower before ovulation than after it. Immediately preceding ovulation the temperature drops about 0.2 degrees, but directly following ovulation the temperature rises about 0.6 degrees (fig. 8.8). There are special thermometers, called basal thermometers, that are calibrated only from 96°–100° so that the tenths-of-degree marks are widely spaced, making it easier to read the small expected changes in temperature. The temperature should be taken immediately upon waking in the morning before leaving bed or starting any activity; and the rectal basal temperature is more accurate than the oral basal temperature.

**SHORT CYCLE**          fertile period

| 1 | 2 | 3 | 4 | 5 | 6 | 7 | 8 | 9 | 10 | 11 | 12 | 13 | 14 | 15 | 16 | 17 | 18 | 19 | 20 | 21 | 22 | 23 | 24 | 25 |
|---|---|---|---|---|---|---|---|---|----|----|----|----|----|----|----|----|----|----|----|----|----|----|----|----|
| 25 | 24 | 23 | 22 | 21 | 20 | 19 | 18 | 17 | 16 | 15 | 14 | 13 | 12 | 11 | 10 | 9 | 8 | 7 | 6 | 5 | 4 | 3 | 2 | 1 |

*days before next cycle* ⟶

**LONG CYCLE**          fertile period

| 1 | 2 | 3 | 4 | 5 | 6 | 7 | 8 | 9 | 10 | 11 | 12 | 13 | 14 | 15 | 16 | 17 | 18 | 19 | 20 | 21 | 22 | 23 | 24 | 25 | 26 | 27 | 28 | 29 |
|---|---|---|---|---|---|---|---|---|----|----|----|----|----|----|----|----|----|----|----|----|----|----|----|----|----|----|----|----|
| 29 | 28 | 27 | 26 | 25 | 24 | 23 | 22 | 21 | 20 | 19 | 18 | 17 | 16 | 15 | 14 | 13 | 12 | 11 | 10 | 9 | 8 | 7 | 6 | 5 | 4 | 3 | 2 | 1 |

*days before next cycle* ⟶

Figure 12.8   According to the rhythm method of birth control, if the shortest period of the year is 25 days and the longest period is 29 days, the fertile period includes day 8 through day 18.

2. The level of sugar in the vagina increases near ovulation. Tes-Tape can be purchased at the drugstore and inserted in the vagina every day. When the yellowish tape turns deepest blue, the sugar level is highest and ovulation is near. The level of acidity can also be tested by the use of pH paper. When the paper shows a change from acid to alkaline, ovulation is near.

3. It's possible to test the stringiness and/or the weight of the cervical mucus. When testing the stringiness, the mucus threads are stretched out the longest at the time of ovulation. When testing the weight by means of a special weighing device, the weight decreases at the time of ovulation.

## Group VI

Douche

**Douching** requires that the vagina and uterus be cleansed with a liquid containing either a commercial product or two tablespoons of vinegar to one quart of water. When a douche is used as a method of birth control, it must be done *immediately* after intercourse.

Although there are no expected side affects, this method is considered unsatisfactory by some because it requires that the woman leave immediately to douch. The pregnancy rate is high (30 or more pregnancies a year per 100 women) because it is almost impossible to douche before some sperm have reached the egg.

These are the only accepted methods of birth control available at the present time. Couples should not rely on other methods suggested by friends, etc.; nor should they believe that single events of intercourse will not result in pregnancy. It is obvious that as long as the egg is present and the sperm have been ejaculated into the vagina, a resultant pregnancy is possible.

## Future Means of Birth Control

After Intercourse

All of the birth control methods discussed require planning ahead, even in the case of coitus interruptus where the male has to be prepared to act promptly. It would be convenient to have a method of birth control that could be used after intercourse has actually occured. Presently, *DES*, a synthetic estrogen, may be given in large doses following intercourse to prevent pregnancy. This is the same drug that formerly was used to prevent miscarriage in some pregnant women. Unfortunately, it has been shown that the daughters of DES-treated women are more apt to develop a rare type of vaginal cancer. The pregnant women received the drug usually from the sixth week through the twelfth week of pregnancy, whereas the after-intercourse, or postcoital pill, is given for only five days.

As a postcoital drug, DES is believed to increase tubular motility so that the embryo arrives early in the uterus when the lining is not properly prepared. Since DES in the large doses required to prevent pregnancy causes nausea and vomiting, it is not usually administered except in cases of rape and incest. Therefore, the search continues for a "morning-after pill." It's possible that prostaglandins might be used for this purpose. **Prostaglandins** are used now to induce abortion because they cause muscle contractions of the uterus and they also cause the corpus luteum to disintegrate. Therefore, taking prostaglandins at the time of expected menstruation would assure the menstrual period.

Immunization Techniques

While some scientists are concerned about the fact that the body is capable of making antibodies against its gametes, others have suggested it as a means of birth control. In other words, it might be possible to purposefully immunize women so that they make antibodies to inactivate their eggs and to immunize men so that they make antibodies to inactivate their sperm. This type of birth control has been studied in animals and found to be reversible after a few cycles. Investigators have also considered using HCGTH as the immunizing agent. Destruction of HCGTH by antibodies would mean that a fertilized egg would never be able to successfully implant itself since the corpus luteum cannot be maintained without active HCGTH. If a woman wished to become pregnant, she could take large doses of HCGTH, overwhelming the antibodies' destructive capacity.

Progesterone

Small doses of progesterone have been found to prevent pregnancy. It may be reasoned that continuously present progesterone inhibits pituitary production of LH so that the corpus luteum never develops. Consequently, there is an inadequate amount of progesterone to prepare the uterine lining for implantation.

Progesterone has been administered as a pill called the "minipill;" injected and implanted for slow release beneath the skin; and incorporated into rings placed in the vagina.

Testosterone

Males who take a synthetic testosterone called danazol fail to make sperm. By the feedback mechanism, the pituitary discontinues production of *FSH* and *ICSH*. Thus, sperm and testosterone are not mady by the testes. It has been found necessary, because of feminizing side effects and low sex drive, to give the male an additional injection of testosterone once a month.

It has also been reported that sertoli cells naturally produce a chemical that inhibits *FSH* production by the pituitary. It is hoped that this chemical might be produced commercially and could therefore be taken in pill form by males.

## Abortions

An **abortion** is the termination of pregnancy before the fetus is capable of survival, presently taken to be a fetal weight of less than one pound. **Spontaneous abortions**, often called **miscarriages**, are those that occur naturally, and **induced abortions** are those that are brought about by external procedures. In most states, induced abortions are now available legally to women who can afford them. The method employed depends on the length of pregnancy.

## Early Abortions

Induced abortions during the first three months of pregnancy are performed either by **dilation** and **curettage** (D and C) or by **uterine aspiration.**

### D and C.

A local or general anesthetic is given and the cervix is dilated by means of a series of cigar-shaped stainless steel dilators of ever-increasing size. A long-handled device with a spoon-shaped end, called a curette, is used to scrape the inside of the uterus.

### Uterine Aspiration.

A local anesthetic is given and the cervix is dilated by using a special vibrator. Uterine contents are sucked out by means of a small metal or plastic tube attached to an aspirator (suction machine). The uterus contracts spontaneously, reducing blood loss. Uterine aspiration is sometimes performed when a woman is 5 to 14 days overdue on menses without definite proof of pregnancy. Under these circumstances, the procedure is called "menstrual regulation" or "menstrual extraction."

## Late Abortions

Induced late abortions are allowed between the sixteenth and twenty-fourth week of pregnancy. After this time, the chances of live birth are considered to be good and therefore such abortions are subject to increased legal control.

The most common method used in the United States for a late abortion is called **salting-out** because it involves the injection of saline (salt solution) or glucose (sugar) solution into the uterus. A quantity of amniotic fluid is removed and replaced by a saline solution. This usually causes the fetus and surrounding membranes to die. Between five and fifty hours later, the uterus begins to contract and the fetus is expelled. The uterus may still have to be cleaned by curettage. Complications such as hemorrhaging and infection are more common with late abortions.

In recent years, prostaglandins have been injected into the amniotic fluid to cause abortion by means of induced uterine contractions. The injection-abortion interval has been shortened to less that twenty hours and there are fewer complications; however, this is a more expensive procedure than salting-out.

# Infertility

In a time when so much attention and emphasis is given to birth control, it is difficult to imagine that for some couples fertility control is no problem. For these individuals, infertility can be a problem that encompasses both emotional and physical aspects. The American Medical Association estimates that 15 percent of all couples in this country are unable to have any children and would therefore be properly termed sterile; another 10 percent have fewer children than they wish and would therefore be properly termed infertile.[2]

Infertility can be due to a number of factors. There may be physiological and structural abnormalities due to genetic inheritance. These could include hormonal imbalance and congenital malformations of the reproductive tract. Diseases such as gonorrhea can cause obstructions of the oviducts and ductus deferentia. And physical traumas, such as radiation and chemical mutagens, can cause chromosomal defects that prevent normal implantation and development. If no medical reason is apparent, it is sometimes felt that infertility might be due to psychological reasons. If so, psychological treatment might be warranted.

## Female Infertility

The two major medical causes for female infertility are failure to ovulate and obstruction of the oviducts. Failure to ovulate may be due to a hormonal imbalance. For example, due to benign tumors of the pituitary some women secrete an excessive amount of lactotropic (prolactin) hormone that is normally only secreted in large amounts following childbirth. These tumors, which interfere with the ability of the pituitary to secrete gonadotropic hormones, can be removed surgically. Also, a drug called bromocriptine can be prescribed; it will bind to the anterior pituitary and inhibit prolactin secretion. At present, however, it is not a recommended treatment of infertility because it is not known whether or not the drug could possibly cause birth defects. Physicians are hopeful, however, that with more data it will be approved as a treatment for infertility.

For women whose infertility does not involve oversecretion of lactotropic hormone, other hormone treatments are available. The drug clomiphene citrate will bind to estrogen receptors on the hypothalamus and cause the hypothalamus to stimulate the pituitary to release FSH and LH. This treatment is often successful. However, if it is not successful, it is possible to administer HMG, a substance extracted from the urine of postmenopausal women, which is rich in FSH and LH. The hypothalamus in postmenopausal women constantly signals the pituitary to release FSH and LH because the ovaries have stopped producing estrogen and progesterone. Most of this FSH and LH are excreted and may be extracted, thereby providing the substance HMG. Unfortunately, HMG can overstimulate the

2. G. B. Kolata, "Infertility: Promising New Treatments,"
   *Science* (13 October 1978): 200.

ovaries and lead to multiple ovulations following the injection of HCGTH (human chorionic gonadotropic hormone, p. 170). If multiple pregnancies result, an abortion may be recommended.

Blocked oviducts can now be reconstructed by a new technique called microsurgery, which is surgery aided by the use of a microscope to magnify the surgical field from 4–25 times. This allows the physician to clearly see the three layers of the tubes and to rejoin each layer separately. The best candidates for microsurgery are women who have had tubal ligation and now wish to have their oviducts rejoined. However, it is possible to cut away obstructions caused by tubal infections and thereafter rejoin the oviducts. Sometimes this leads to tubal pregnancies because the fertilized egg is prevented from reaching the uterus. Women with inoperative damaged oviducts could possibly become pregnant by means of in vitro fertilization and subsequent implantation. This extremely new and experimental procedure is discussed on page 171.

Male Infertility

Males can be treated for hormonal imbalance and physical obstruction of the ductus deferentia in the same manner as females. Gonadotropic hormone treatment and microsurgery could possibly lead to a normal sperm count. In addition, varicocoele, swollen veins in the scrotum, is a primary cause of male infertility. It too can be cured surgically.

If no medical reason can be found and the sperm count is low, then it is possible to concentrate the sperm and use this concentrate to artifically inseminate the wife. Artificial insemination is further discussed on page 170. If the quantity of sperm is considered adequate, it's possible that the quality is inadequate. The quality of sperm is determined by microscopic examination of an ejaculate. Men with a large number of immotile or abnormally shaped sperm may be infertile. Odd-shaped sperm are believed to be an indication of defective chromosomes. But since there are so many uncertainties as to what constitutes a normal sperm count and normal sperm appearance, some investigators feel that the best course of action is to concentrate on correcting female infertility.

---

## Summary

Devices and procedures used to prevent conception are divided into six categories. In the first group, sterilization refers to vasectomy in the male and tubal ligation in the female. The pill, which usually contains both estrogen and progesterone, prevents ovulation due to feedback control over the anterior pituitary. Group II and III includes the IUD, diaphragm, and condom. The IUD may prevent implantation, while the latter two prevent conception. Group IV and V include coitus interruptus, the rhythm method, and intravaginal foams, creams, and jellies. Coitus interruptus is the withdrawal of the penis before ejaculation. The rhythm method of birth control allows intercourse only on "safe" days. Determining these "safe days" is more successful if the woman uses the basal temperature method rather than the calendar method. Insertion of vaginal foam is more effective than jellies and creams. Douching, or rinsing out the vagina following intercourse, is an old but not very effective means of birth control. Since all these methods have some drawbacks, research progressess to find a morning after, once a month, or long-lasting birth control procedure. If an unwanted pregnancy does occur, an abortion is sometimes performed. Early abortion procedures, especially uterine aspiration, is preferred over late abortions requiring salting-out or prostaglandin injection.

Some couples are infertile and do not have as many children as they wish. Infertility can sometimes be cured by gonadotropic hormonal treatment or surgical treatment especially to repair damaged oviducts in the female and damaged ductus deferentia or swollen scrotal veins in the male.

## Terms

| | |
|---|---|
| coitus interruptus | intrauterine device (IUD) |
| condom | prostaglandin |
| curettage (curette) | spermicidal |
| diaphragm | sterilization |
| douche | tubal ligation |
| infertility | vasectomy |

## Review

1. State nine means of birth control and rate the effectiveness of each.
2. Which types of birth control measures require operative procedures? Why don't these operations affect the secondary sex characteristics?
3. Which birth control devices must be fitted and/or prescribed by a physician?
4. Which types of birth control devices may be purchased in a drug store with no doctor's prescription? Of these, which is the most effective?
5. Which is the "natural" means of birth control? Theoretically, how does the natural method work? Explain its high failure rate.
6. Name three means of birth control that are being perfected at this time. Explain how each theoretically works.
7. What are the two types of abortion? Which type is safest?
8. What are some treatments for female infertility? For male infertility?

# Venereal Disease                                                  13

**Venereal diseases** (VD), unlike genetic diseases, are contagious diseases that are usually sexually transmitted directly from one person to another. The microorganisms that cause VD, as listed in chart 13.1, are bacteria (gonorrhea, syphilis, chancroid); viruses (herpes genitalis); fungus (vaginitis); and microorganisms intermediate between viruses and bacteria (granuloma venereum, lymphogranuloma venereum, urethritis). Figure 13.1 gives a diagrammatic representation of these organisms, all of which are microscopic; in fact, viruses cannot be seen without the aid of the electron microscope.

When microorganisms invade the body, they multiply rapidly. Being **parasitic**, they depend on nutrients supplied by the body while their waste products and toxic by-products have a destructive influence on the body's tissues. Of course, viruses are small enough to invade the cells themselves and in this way bring about cellular destruction. The body attempts to ward off infection in two ways: certain white cells engulf the microorganisms (fig. 13.2) and certain other white cells sometimes produce antibodies (fig. 13.3). Pus, which may appear at the site of an infection, is made up of dead white cells, dead and living microorganisms, and cellular debris.

If, in response to an infection, adequate antibody production begins, the individual is thereafter *immune* to this infection and will never again have this illness. Antibodies are specific, however, and a new and different type is needed for each infective agent. For illnesses in which immunity is possible, vaccination is often possible. Vaccines contain treated or dead microorganisms that, when injected, cause the production of antibodies without causing the illness.

Unfortunately, humans cannot develop immunity to gonorrhea and syphilis, the two most commonly reported venereal diseases. We are not surprised, then, that these two contagious diseases, which can be contracted time and time

## Chart 13.1
Venereal Diseases

| Name | Organism | Resultant Condition | Treatment |
|---|---|---|---|
| *Transmitted by Sexual Intercourse* | | | |
| *Gonorrhea | Gonococcus (bacterium) | Adult: sterility due to scarring of epididymis and tubes Rarely: septicemia Newborn: blindness | Penicillin injections Tetracycline tablets Eye drops (silver nitrate or penicillin) |
| *Syphilis | Treponema pallidum (bacterium) | Adult: gummas, cardiovascular neurosyphilis Newborn: congenital syphilis (abnormalities and blindness) | Penicillin injections Tetracycline tablets |
| **Chancroid (soft chancre) | Hemophilus ducrey (bacterium) | Chancres, bubos | Tetracycline Sulfa drugs |
| *Not Necessarily Transmitted by Sexual Intercourse* | | | |
| *Urethritis (NGU) in men | Various microorganisms | Clean discharge | Tetracycline |
| *Vaginitis | Trichomonas (protozoan) | Frothy white or yellow discharge | Metronidazole |
| | Candida albicans (yeast) | Thick, white, curdy discharge (moniliasis) | Nystatin |
| **Lymphogranuloma venereum (LGV) | Microorganism | Ulcerating bubos Rectal stricture | Tetracycline Sulfa drugs |
| **Granuloma venereum (inguinal) | Donovania granulomatis | Raw, open, extended sore | Tetracycline |
| Venereal warts | Virus | Warts | Podophyllin |
| *Genital herpes | Herpes simplex virus | Sores | Palliative treatment |
| *Crabs | Arthropod | Itching | Gamma benzene hexachloride |

*Of fairly common occurrence.    **More common in warmer climates.

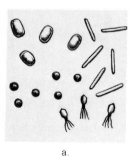 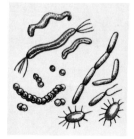 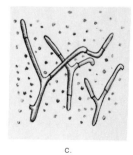

a.    b.    c.

Figure 13.1    Microorganisms. (a) virus, (b) bacteria, and (c) fungi.

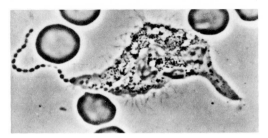

Figure 13.2   White cell ingesting a chain of streptococcal bacteria. (Source: Public Affairs Division, Pfizer, Inc., 235 E. 42nd Street, New York, NY 10017.)

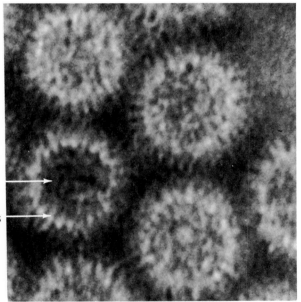

**viruses**

**antibodies**

Figure 13.3   An electron micrograph that shows antibodies (light areas) attached to viruses (dark areas). (Source: Almeida, J.D., Cinader, B., and Howatson, A.F., The Structure of Antigen-Antibody Complexes, A Study of Electron Microscopy *Journal of Experimental Medicine*, 118: 327–340, 1963 by copyright permission of The Rockefeller University Press.)

again, are quite prevalent. Figure 13.4 indicates that gonorrhea is by far the most commonly reported infectious disease in the United States. No wonder it is said that we are presently having a VD epidemic.

Presently, the only mechanism available to control venereal disease is prompt and proper treatment. Persons who find that they have venereal disease must tell their sexual contacts so that they, too, can be examined and treated. Self-diagnosis and self-treatment are usually inadequate, and all those who believe they have venereal disease should receive proper medical care.

For each venereal disease discussed below, we will consider (1) the earliest sign of infection, usually a visible external response to infection, (2) the internal effects or response to infection, and (3) the final resultant condition if treatment has been delayed. Chart 13.1 lists these resultant conditions and gives the antibiotic drug of choice for treatment.

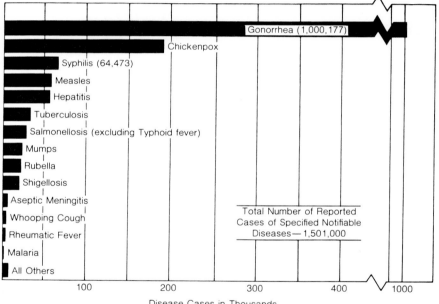

Figure 13.4   The number of reported cases of gonococcal infections reported in 1973. Since the majority of cases probably went unreported, the actual total may have exceeded 2.5 million. (Source: U.S. Public Health Service.)

Human Reproduction

# Major Venereal Diseases
Gonorrhea

**Gonorrhea**, which is much more apt to be diagnosed earlier in the male than the female, develops as follows:

*External Response (a few days after exposure):*

**Males:** painful urination accompanied by a continuous discharge, which may be clear but is more often white or yellow green and purulent due to presence of pus (fig. 13.5).

**Females:** most females are asymptomatic (have no symptoms). A discharge at the cervix goes unrecognized (fig. 13.6). Painful urination is possible but not common.

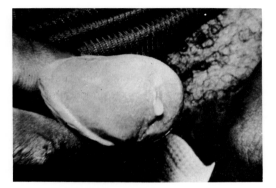

Figure 13.5   Gonorrhea in the male can be recognized by a greenish-yellow discharge. (Source: HEW, Public Health Service, Center for Disease Control, Atlanta, GA.)

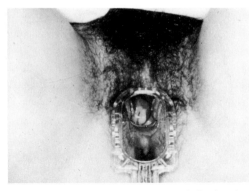

Figure 13.6   Identification of gonorrhea in the female requires internal examination. (Source: HEW, Public Health Service, Center for Disease Control, Atlanta, GA.)

*Internal Response (a few weeks or months after exposure):*

**Males:** infection of the glands, including the prostrate, along the path of the urethra may cause difficult urination and lower pelvic pain.

**Females:** PID (pelvic inflammatory disease) occurs after the bacteria move through the uterus at the time of menstruation to the tubes. Menstrual difficulties and a temperature may be present.

*Resultant Condition:*

**Males:** infection of epididymis causes scrotum to be red, hot, and painful. STERILITY occurs due to the build-up of scar tissue in the epididymis.

**Females:** infection of the tubes, called **salpingitis,** may require exploratory abdominal surgery for proper diagnosis. STERILITY occurs due to the build-up of scar tissue in the Fallopian tubes.

*Discussion.* Most males seek early treatment due to infection of the urethra causing painful urination. Usually, the physician can determine that gonorrhea is the cause, but to be certain a sample of the discharge should be examined microscopically (fig. 13.7) to reveal the gonorrhea gonococcus. Also, the discharge may be spread on a culture plate (fig. 13.8) and gonorrhea colonies will grow, confirming the diagnosis. Unfortunately, the female usually lacks symptoms until the disease is well advanced. However, her discharge can also be examined and tested to confirm her condition. Therefore, a male having gonorrhea should be sure to tell all his partners so that they might be diagnosed and treated.

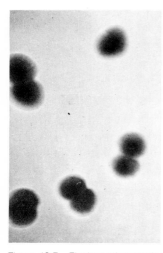

Figure 13.7 Electron micrograph of *Neisseria gonorrhea,* the bacteria that causes gonorrhea.

Human Reproduction

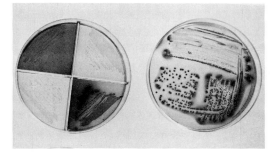

Figure 13.8   Culture plate with bacterial colonies.

Homosexual males develop gonorrhea proctitis, or infection of the anus, for which the symptoms are pain in the anus and blood or pus in the feces. Oral sex can cause infection of the throat (pharyngitis) and tonsillitis. These conditions should receive the same antibiotic therapy recommended for gonorrhea.

If a pregnant woman has gonorrhea gonococcus present in the vagina, her newborn child will be exposed to the bacteria during its passage through the birth canal. There is a resultant bacterial infection of the eyes leading to blindness. Because of this, all newborn infants receive eye drops containing tetracycline or penicillin as a protective measure.

Very rarely, the gonorrhea gonococcus invades the bloodstream. The term **septicemia** refers to any bacterial infection present in the blood circulatory system. Within a week of the beginning of septicemia, the joints become swollen, red, and painful and antibiotic therapy must be given promptly to avoid permanent injury.

Syphilis

Syphilis is caused by a type of bacterium called a **spirochete** (fig. 13.9). Because this bacteria cannot be stained, it shows up only when viewed on a dark-field microscope. Such microscopes are not routinely available and so a blood test is the usual test for syphilis. The blood tests, of which there are several, all rely on detecting the presence of antibodies to syphilis, rather than the presence of the organism itself. Syphilis is less common than gonorrhea, but it is the more serious of the two infections.

*External Response:*

Primary Stage: 10 days to 3 months

A hard **chancre** (ulcerated sore with hard edges) indicates the site of infection. The chancre will heal by itself (fig. 13.10).

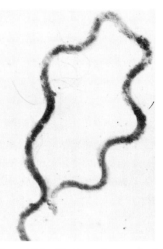

Figure 13.9 Electron micrograph of *Treponema pallidum*, the bacteria that causes syphilis.

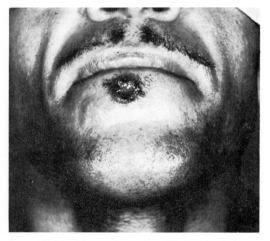

Figure 13.10 Primary stage of syphilis is a hard chancre, shown here on the lip. (Source: HEW, Public Health Service, Center for Disease Control, Atlanta, GA.)

*Internal Response:*

Secondary Stage: 2 weeks to 6 months

A **skin rash** that does not itch (fig. 13.11) appears on the body including the palms of the hands and soles of the feet. There may be hair loss and

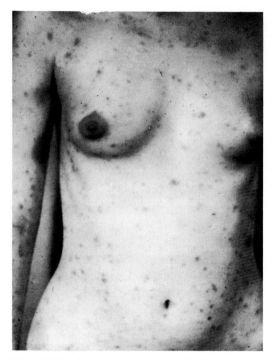

Figure 13.11   Secondary stage of syphilis is a body rash.
(Source: HEW, Public Health Service, Center for Disease
Control, Atlanta, GA.)

gray patches on the mucous membranes. These symptoms also disappear of their own accord.

Latent Stage: 1 year to death

Syphilis has been temporarily brought under control by the body itself. The person is noninfectious and has no symptoms.

*Resultant Condition:*

Tertiary Stage:

(a) Benign (3 to 7 years): **Gummas** (fig. 13.12), which are large, destructive ulcers, appear on the skin and within the internal organs.

(b) Cardiovascular (10 to 40 years): The heart and blood vessels in particular are attacked by the microorganism.

(c) Neurosyphilis (10 to 20 years): The spinal cord and brain are attacked by the microorganism. Insanity is the end result.

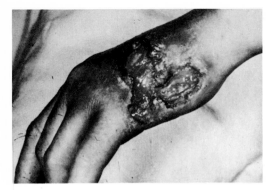

Figure 13.12  Tertiary stage of syphilis is gummas, shown here on the hand. (Source: HEW, Public Health Service, Center for Disease Control, Atlanta, GA.)

*Discussion.*  Septicemia is always present with syphilis. The spirochete always invades the bloodstream and organs of the individual. Because the first two stages of syphilis disappear of their own accord, the individual may believe that he has been cured, but this is far from true. The disease is simply awaiting the time when it can become active and more damaging. Syphilis can be cured even if it has reached the tertiary stage, so a person should never feel that it is too late for treatment.

*Congenital syphilis.*  Syphilis can be passed from mother to child, usually when the disease is in its primary or secondary stage. The infant is born with all sorts of possible structural abnormalities and may be blind. If the newborn survives infancy, the child has characteristic teeth, called Hutchinson's teeth.

Genital Herpes

This condition manifests itself when the vagina, cervix, vulva, or urethra in women and the penis and urethra in men tingles and burns about 2–20 days after contact. External and internal blisters appear but soon rupture to produce painful shallow lesions (fig. 13.13). These symptoms may be accompanied by fever, pain upon urination, and swollen lymph nodes. Although all symptoms tend to disappear after 10–14 days, they can recur without further sexual contact. Since recurrent genital herpes is common, it is believed that this disease may be second to gonorrhea as the most prevalent venereal disease in the United States. Infection of the newborn can occur.

Genital herpes is caused by *herpes simplex virus* of which there are two types; *Type 1* usually causes cold sores and fever blisters while *Type 2* causes genital herpes. Several studies have shown a definite connection between genital herpes and cancer of the cervix and prostate, although it has not been proven that the herpes virus actually causes the cancer.

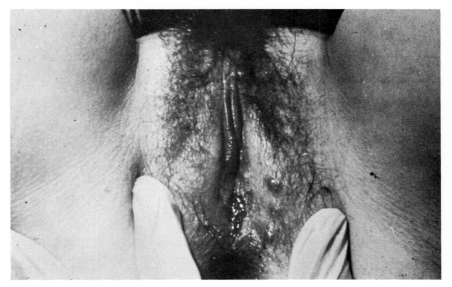

Figure 13.13.   Herpes Simplex affecting the vulva. (Source: HEW.)

## Lesser Venereal Diseases

Chancroid

*External Response (1 to 5 days):*

> **Soft chancres** (an oozing ulcer with soft edges) increase in number on the external genitalia.

*Internal Response (3 to 6 days):*
Infection of the lymph nodes in the groin causes them to swell and become painful.

*Resultant Condition (5 to 8 days):*
Lymph nodes may fuse to form a **bubo** and ulcerate, causing a large, open sore.

Lymphogranuloma venereum (LGV)

*External response (5 to 21 days):*
A pimplelike sore marks the site of infection.

*Internal Response (10 to 30 days):*
Infection of the lymph nodes in the groin causes them to swell and become painful (fig. 13.14).

*Resultant Condition:*
Lymph nodes may fuse to form a bubo and ulcerate, causing a large, open sore.

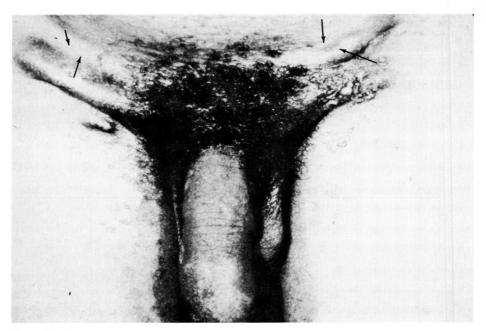

Figure 13.14 *Lymphogranuloma venereum* is a venereal disease characterized by infected lymph nodes. (Source: HEW.)

*Discussion.* To distinguish between these two infections, remember that they are caused by different organisms. Chancroid is caused by a bacterium, while LGV is caused by a microorganism intermediate between a virus and bacteria. Also, the chancroid is primarily a disease characterized by external sores, while LGV is primarily characterized by bubos, leading to external abcesses. LGV is an infection of the **lymphatic system**, which consists of lymph veins that drain fluid from the tissues and lymph nodes that fight infection. If the lymph vessels are blocked due to infection, the genital organs can swell, causing elephantiasis (fig. 13.15). Also, the infection can spread by way of the lymph vessels to the anus. The walls of the anus will narrow, forming a rectal stricture that must be corrected by surgery.

Urethritis in the Male and Vaginitis in the Female

Males may have a discharge and painful urination due to infection with other organisms beside gonococcus. This is called nongonococcal urethritis (NGU). The causative organisms are various.

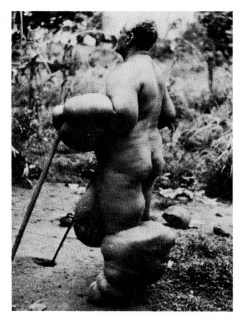

Figure 13.15   A person with elephantiasis experiences
extreme swelling of body parts due to blocked lymph vessels.
(Source: Markell, E.K. and Voge, M., *Medical Parasitology*, 4th
ed. W.B. Saunders, Philadelphia.)

Females very often have **vaginitis**, or infection of the vagina, caused by
the protozoan *trichomonas* or the yeast, *Candida albicans*. The protozoan
infection causes a frothy white or yellow discharge accompanied by itching, while
the yeast infection causes a thick, white, curdy discharge accompanied by itching.
Both of these infections can occur without sexual intercourse. Trichomonas can
be contracted from infected towels and washcloths, for example. Candida
albicans, however, is a normal organism found in the vagina; its growth simply
increases beyond normal under certain circumstances. Women taking the birth
control pill have been prone to yeast infections, for example.

Granuloma Venereum

Granuloma venereum (fig. 13.16) is an infection of the external genitalia
with no internal response. A painless bump or blister becomes an open sore
that is raised, rounded, velvety, and bleeds easily. The infected area may cover
the external genitalia and extend to the thighs, lower abdomen, and buttocks,
making the whole area red and raw.

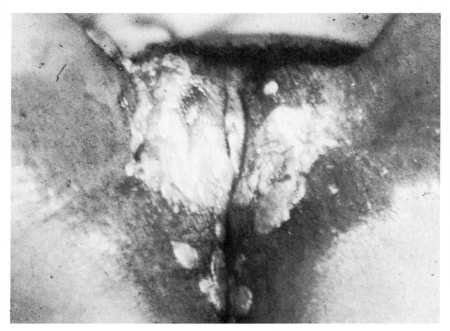

Figure 13.16  *Granuloma venereum.* (Source: HEW.)

### Virus Conditions

*Warts.*   Warts may appear on the genitals (fig. 13.17)—the glans penis and foreskin in males and the vaginal opening in females are common locations. Venereal warts vary in appearance from pink or red and soft with an indented, cauliflowerlike appearance to small, hard, and yellow-gray resembling ordinary warts.

### Crabs

Small lice, that look like crabs under the microscope (fig. 13.18), infect the pubic and underarm hair of humans. The females lay their eggs around the base of the hair and these eggs hatch within a few days to produce a large number of animals that suck blood from their host and cause itching.

Crabs can be contracted by direct contact with an infected person or by contact with his/her clothing or bedding. Self-treatment is possible as proper, effective medication may be purchased without a doctor's prescription.

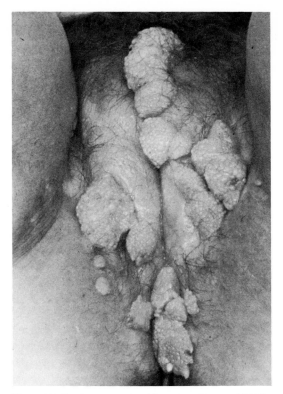

Figure 13.17 Genital warts of the vulva. (Source: HEW.)

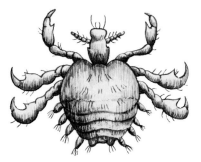

Figure 13.18 *Phthirus pubis*, the parasitic louse that infects the pubic hair of humans.

## Summary

Chart 13.1 lists the venereal diseases discussed in this chapter. In the United States, gonorrhea and syphilis, which are caused by bacterial infections, are believed by some to be the most prevalent sexually transmitted diseases. It has been suggested, however, that genital herpes, which is caused by a viral infection, might be just as prevalent. Gonorrhea is more easily detected in the male because of painful urination; the female is often asymptomatic. Even so, eventual sterility is possible in both sexes. Syphilis, which has three stages (chancre, rash, gummas), can end in cardiovascular and brain impairment. Genital herpes is simply small, painful external and internal ulcers. A newborn infant can acquire gonorrhea infection of the eyes and herpes infection of the body as it passes through the birth canal. Syphilis is acquired prenatally and causes birth defects.

Other diseases such as chancroid, lymphogranuloma, and granuloma venereum are not common in this country. Nonspecific urethritis is common in men as is vaginitis in females.

## Terms

| | |
|---|---|
| antibody | Hutchinson's teeth |
| buboes | immunity |
| chancre | microorganism |
| congenital syphilis | septicemia |
| *Gonorrhea gonococcus* | *Treponema pallidum* |
| gumma | *Trichomonas* |
| herpes simplex virus | |

## Review

1. What is the normal method by which the body fights infection? Are these methods effective against venereal disease?
2. What is the external, internal, and resultant effect of gonorrhea in the male and female?
3. What is the test and the cure for gonorrhea? Is self-diagnosis possible? Is self-treatment possible?
4. What is the external, internal, and resultant effect of syphilis?
5. What is the test and cure for syphilis? Is self-diagnosis possible? Is self-treatment possible?
6. How might these two venereal diseases affect the unborn and/or newborn?

7. What are the two primary causes of vaginitis in the female?

8. Distinguish between chancroid, lymphogranuloma venereum, and granuloma venereum.

9. What two infections of the genitals can be caused by viruses?

10. "Crabs" is caused by what type of animal? How do you get crabs?

11. If you should happen to contract a venereal disease, what should be done, step-by-step?

---

## Further Readings for Part 2

The Boston Women's Health Book Collective. 1976. *Our Bodies, Ourselves: A Book by and for Women*, 2nd ed. New York: Simon & Schuster.

Edwards, R.G. 1970. Human embryos in the laboratory. *Scientific American* 223(10):44–54.

Gagon, John H. 1977. *Human Sexualities*. Glenview, Ill.: Scott, Foresman and Co.

Goldstein, B. 1976. *Human Sexuality*. New York: McGraw-Hill Book Company, Inc.

Guttmacher, A.F. 1973. *Pregnancy, Birth and Family Planning*. New York: Viking Press.

Katchadourian, H. 1977. *The Biology of Adolescence*. San Francisco: W.H. Freeman & Co.

Katchadourian, H.A., and Lunde, D.T. 1972. *Fundamentals of Human Sexuality*. New York: Holt, Rinehart and Winston.

Masters, W.H., and Johnson, V.E. 1966. *Human Sexual Response*. Boston: Little, Brown and Co.

Moore, J.A. 1972. *Heredity and Development*, 2nd ed. New York: Oxford University Press.

Page, E.W., et al. 1976. *Human Reproduction*, 2nd ed. Philadelphia: W.B. Saunders Co.

Rugh, R., and Shettles, L.B. 1971. *From Conception to Birth: The Drama of Life's Beginnings*. New York: Harper & Row, Publishers.

Taussig, H.B. 1962. The thalidomide syndrome. *Scientific American* 207 (2) August, 29–35.

Wilson, S., et al. 1977. *Human Sexuality*. New York: West Publishing Co.

Vander, A.J., et al. 1975. *Human Physiology*. New York: McGraw-Hill Book Company, Inc.

Volpe, Peter E. 1979. *Man, Nature and Society,* 2nd ed. Dubuque, Iowa: Wm. C. Brown Company Publishers.

# Part 3 Evolution, Behavior, and Population

# Evolution of Sexual Reproduction

# 14

Sexual reproduction evolved or came into being during the course of the history of the earth. The first cell, believed to be a product of chemical evolution, simply divided to produce daughter cells. This type of asexual reproduction (fig. 14.1) is common to bacteria today. Bacteria are haploid and it may have been that the first cell was also haploid, meaning that it had only one set of genes. Such a life cycle seems inadequate for two reasons: (1) genetic variation is solely dependent on mutation, and (2) any faulty gene must express itself since the adult is haploid. For bacteria the system works well however, because numerous bacteria come into existence within a relatively short period of time. This means that actually the mutation rate is high, and a few defective genes will not reduce the total number of bacteria significantly.

Evolution

Through the evolutionary process, sexual reproduction evolved from asexual reproduction. Evolution, the process by which new types of organisms come into being, requires a considerable length of time because it depends on genetic variations (genotype changes) that are of benefit to the organism. Such variations enhance the likelihood of the organism's survival. "Survival of the fittest" does not mean that the "fit" personally destroy the "nonfit." Rather, the fit are more

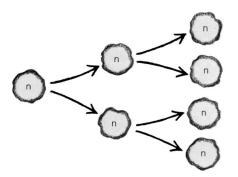

Figure 14.1   In asexual reproduction there is only one parent and the offspring have the same genotype as the parent.

likely to survive and reproduce and pass on their genes to the next generation. What type of genetic variation is apt to make an organism more fit? A simple illustration of this is given in figure 14.2. Variations that cause the organism to be more adapted to the environment are those that increase the possibility of survival. Thus they are the ones that are more likely to be passed on. "Adapted" means that the organism's physical, physiological, and even behavioral characteristics are suited to the environment. The physical, physiological, and behavioral characteristics that enable a fish to survive in water are those that make it suited or adapted to its environment. These are the features or adaptations that will allow a fish to survive and pass on its genes.

Evolution is a continuous natural process in which certain genotypes are passed on to the next generation to a greater extent than other genotypes. These genotypes have been "selected"; hence, the process is called *natural*

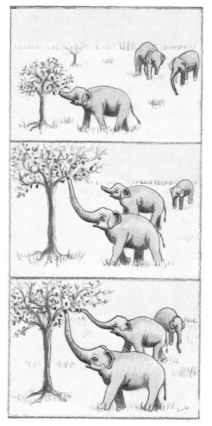

Figure 14.2  Adaptation by natural selection is illustrated by this hypothetical example in which elephants with long trunks are more fit because of a change in the environment.

Evolution, Behavior, and Population

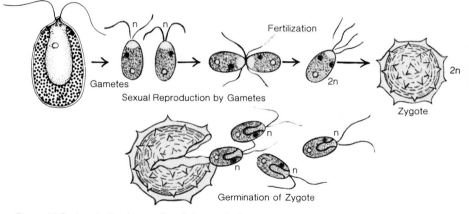

Figure 14.3  In primitive forms of sexual reproduction, exemplified by *Chlamydomonas,* the adult is haploid, the gametes look alike, the zygote overwinters, and meiosis produces new individuals with a different genotype than the parent. (After Mader, *Inquiry into Life*, 2d edition.)

*selection.* The genotypes that caused better adaptation to the environment are the ones that are selected; these are the ones that are passed on to the next generation because of unequal reproduction.

Sexual Reproduction

Sexual reproduction (reproduction by means of gametes) is first seen in primitive organisms that have a life cycle similar to that in figure 14.3. In this life cycle, typically, the zygote "overwinters," meaning that it has a hard protective covering that allows survival during the cold winter months. It may be theorized that this was an advantage favorable to the continuance of sexual reproduction. In this life cycle, there is also routine genetic variation because the offspring never has the same genes as either parent; instead, the offspring has a different combination of genes. Thus, sexual reproduction gives another method of achieving genetic variation in addition to chance mutation. Obviously, this increases the potential for possible adaptation, and sexual reproduction has become almost universal among living organisms.

The life cycle depicted in figure 14.3, however, still has a haploid adult due to the fact that meiosis occurs after formation of the zygote. A diploid adult is preferred because with a double set of genes a defective gene may be masked or dominated by an effective gene. It is not surprising, then, that in the most advanced cycles, the adult is diploid (fig. 14.4).

*Plants.*  Higher plants have a life cycle that includes a diploid adult and sexual reproduction. Most higher plants have flowers (fig. 14.5) in which there are male

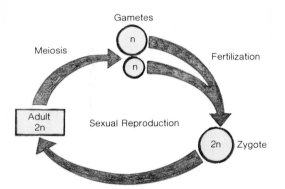

Figure 14.4 In advanced forms of sexual reproduction, the adult is diploid, meiosis produces the gametes, and the diploid zygote becomes the adult.

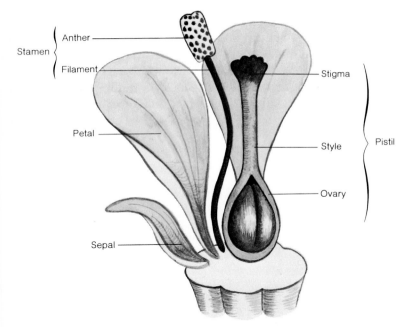

Figure 14.5 Diagram of a flower. The pistil is the female part of a flower and the stamen is the male part.

and female parts. The male parts of a flower, the stamens, have a portion called the anther, which produces pollen. A pollen grain contains the male gamete, the sperm nucleus. The female part of the flower, called the pistil, includes an expanded portion, the ovary, that contains the ovules, each of which produces an egg. The manner in which the sperm nucleus reaches the egg in plants is an adaptation to life on land.

*Land environment.* While it seems almost ridiculous to say that water is wet and land is dry, this very fact is the dramatic environmental difference between life in the water and life on land. Life arose in the water because a water environment is less hazardous to living things. Cells are more than 50 percent water and are in constant danger of desiccation, or drying out, in a dry environment. Any organism living on the land must have a means of reproduction that prevents desiccation of the gametes and the zygote.

In plants, the hard outer covering of a pollen grain protects the sperm nucleus from drying out. In addition, a pollen grain is windblown or carried by insects to the top of the pistil. In other words, through the evolutionary process, reproduction in plants is not dependent on swimming sperm. This is advantageous because plants lack locomotion and male and female cannot get together for procreation as animals do.

*Animals.* The life cycle of animals, shown in figure 14.4, is the most advanced life cycle. Gametogenesis produces the gametes, the only haploid portion of the cycle. Since each parent contributes only half its genes to the zygote, the zygote has a different combination of genes than either parent. The adult is diploid and has a double set of genes.

Some animals are adapted to reproduction in the water and some are adapted to reproduction on the land. To illustrate the differences between reproduction in water and reproduction on land, consider the manner in which frogs reproduce (fig. 14.6) as compared to reproduction in humans. The male frog lacks a penis and simply clasps the female during amplexus, causing her to release her eggs in the water. Thereafter, the male releases his sperm. Fertilization occurs externally in the water and the zygote develops into the swimming embryo (the tadpole) externally in the water.

In contrast, the human male has a penis and deposits the sperm inside the female. Fertilization occurs internally, protecting the swimming sperm from the possibility of drying out. The zygote develops inside the female; consequently, the embryo is also protected from desiccation. The anatomical and physiological manner in which humans reproduce is an adaptation to life on land. Is there reproductive behavior also adaptive or suited to the passage of the genes from one generation to another? The new science of sociobiology maintains not only that the genotype determines behavior, but also that the evolutionary process has selected those behavioral traits that assure that the genotype will be passed on. It stands to reason that those individuals adapted to assuring the passage of their genes will indeed be those individuals who do so.

In the next section, we will first explore the tenet that behavioral patterns do evolve; then, we will examine the behavioral traits of baboons and men to see if these behavioral traits seem to be adapted toward assuring passage of the genes.

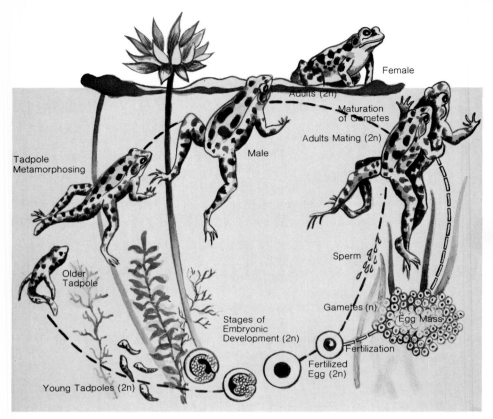

Figure 14.6 Reproduction in water is illustrated by the life cycle of a frog. (Source: *Biology: An Inquiry into the Nature of Life* by Stanley L. Weinberg. © Copyright 1977 by Allyn and Bacon, Inc. Reproduced by permission.)

## Genes and Behavior

One example of behavioral evolution is the nest-building habits of the parrot, *Agapornis* (fig. 14.7). Three species of this genus have different methods of building nests. Females of the most primitive species use their sharp bills for cutting bits of bark, which they carry in their feathers to a site where they make a pad or a nest. Females of a more advanced species cut long regular strips of material, which are placed for transport only in the rump feathers. These strips are used to make elaborate nests with a special section for the eggs. Females of the most advanced species carry stronger materials, such as sticks, in their beaks. They construct roofed nests with two chambers and a passageway. The steady progression here from primitive to advanced suggests that an evolution of behavioral patterns has taken place.

Evolution, Behavior, and Population

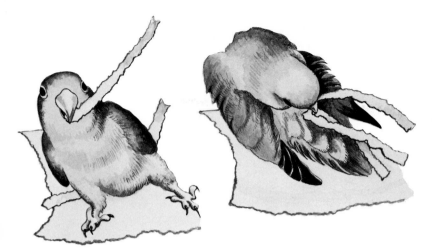

Figure 14.7 *Agapornis* parrots. Cut strips of paper (left) and then tuck them into rump feathers (right). (Source: After William C. Dilger Photos).

The fact that genes are controlling these traits can be supported by the following experiment. The species that carries material in its rump feathers has been mated to the species that carries material in the beak. The resulting hybrid birds cut strips and try to tuck them in their rump feathers but are unsuccessful. It is as if the genes of one parent require them to tuck the strips, but the genes of the other species prevents them from succeeding.

An example that behavior is adapted for continuance of the genotype is found among the black-headed gulls, who always remove broken eggshells from their nests after the young have hatched. In a series of experiments, investigators determined that nests with broken shells remaining were subject to more predator attack than those from which shells had been removed. It can be reasoned that gulls that remove broken eggshells and other conspicuous objects from their nests will successfully raise more young than gulls that do not do so. This behavior pattern may have been selected through the evolutionary process because it improved reproductive success.

Mammals

Mammals differ from other vertebrates (chart 14.1) in that the embryo develops within the uterus of the female. The behavior of mammals may very well be adapted to this situation and the genes may dictate behavior that is consistent with this anatomical fact.

Females produce many fewer eggs than males produce sperm. This difference in gamete production is not a disadvantage to females because they have the assurance that the offspring is theirs—an assurance that males never

**Chart 14.1**
Vertebrates

| Class | Example | Development |
|---|---|---|
| Fish | Perch, Trout, Haddock | In water |
| Amphibian | Frog, Salamander | In water |
| Reptile | Snake, Turtle | Hard-shall egg on land |
| Bird | Chicken, Penquin | Hard-shell egg on land |
| Mammal | Horse, Elephant, Ape, Human | Within uterus of mother |

have. Lacking physiological certainty, it behooves males to attempt to impregnate as many females as possible. This, obviously, is common among nonhuman species. On the other hand, since females need the protection of males, it seems consistent that they would be faithful. This difference in the sexes is commonly expressed in the statement—males have more sexual freedom than females.

Females usually care for the young that were borne by them and definitely carry one-half of their genes. Males may not contribute as greatly to the care of the young because they have no physiological evidence that the offspring belongs to them and that it carries one-half of their genes. Since females need protection while they care for their offspring, they may have tended to select aggressive males on which to be dependent. The evolutionary outcome is that females would be docile and subservient while males would be combatant and dominant.

Thus far, we have been simply reasoning as to what behavioral patterns seem to be consistent with the anatomical facts. We might see if this reasoning holds true by examining the behavioral patterns of baboons and humans.

Baboons

The baboon male weighs about 70 pounds and is about 35 inches tall, while the female is about 30 pounds and 20 inches tall. One interesting explanation for this extreme difference in size is that it is the most economical way to achieve protection while limiting food consumption.

Baboons that live in the plains of Africa (fig. 14.8) may be attacked by jackals, hyenas, lions, cheetahs, and leopards, but these animals rarely succeed in killing a baboon because of the ferocity of the baboon male. The males are formidable not only because of their size but also because of their disposition and their long, sharp canine teeth (fig. 14.9). When necessary, they sink their teeth into an attacker and tear out a hunk of flesh. A troop of baboons is very dependent on the males to fight off would-be predators, and most observers report that the males never fail in this responsibility.

Evolution, Behavior, and Population

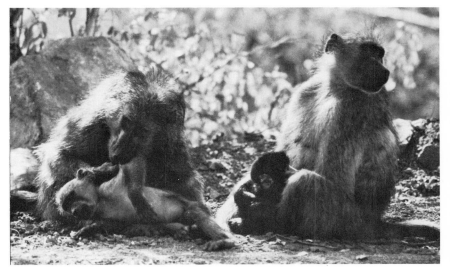

Figure 14.8 Among baboons females care for the young.
(Source: photo courtesy of South African Tourist Corp.)

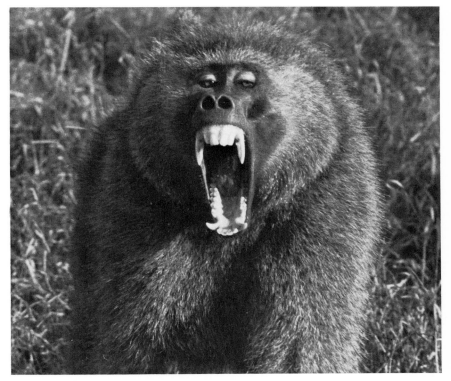

Figure 14.9 Male baboon displaying full threat. (Source: Irven
DeVore/Anthro-Photo.)

Males are competitive and aggressive, but among troop members this aggression is controlled by the social constraints of dominance (fig. 14.10). Each baboon knows his or her place in a hierarchy, and dominance is established by psychological contests between individuals in which it is determined who will conceed. When females are in estrus (heat) and able to conceive, they seek out the company of the dominant males. During this time, the female's position in the troop is elevated as the males keep company with her. Following copulation, pregnancy lasts for about six months. The mother takes care of the birth herself and travels with the troop on the day of the birth. The newborn baboon is capable of clinging to the underside of its mother, where it nurses. The first day or so, the mother may assist the infant by holding a hand on it. Since this tends to slow her progress, a dominant male may drop back and walk with her, stopping when she stops and generally looking after her.

Males seem to be very interested in the newborn and especially watch over infants and youngsters when the troop is on the move. Should a youngster be stranded when the troop is under attack, a male will quickly snatch it up and return it to its mother.

Baboon behavior seems to be consistent with the description of mammalian division of labor described earlier. Females care for the young and are dependent on aggressive males. The baboons live in troops in which more than one male is available to protect the whole group. Several males mate with the same female, but then they have access to all the females. The aggressiveness of the male baboons is held in check by the troop's practice of dominance.

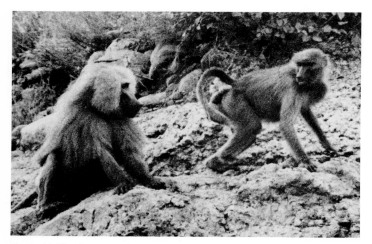

Figure 14.10   A baboon presenting to a more dominant baboon. (Source: Hans Kummer.)

Evolution, Behavior, and Population

## Humans

According to sociobiologists who have extended the theory of the evolution of sexual behavior to humans, males have traditionally been valued for their position in the world and females for their ability to reproduce. Young women are apt to marry older males because they are capable of providing for a family while the young woman is capable of producing offspring.

Humans are the only mammal lacking an estrus; the female is continuously amenable to sexual intercourse. Could this possibly be an adaptation to the necessities of reproduction? Human infants are helpless and require the committed attention of at least one parent, usually the woman. The mother and child need the protection of the father for an extended length of time (fig. 14.11). The fact that sex is continuously available may help assure a continued relationship between male and female as they both contribute to the upbringing of the offspring.

Males tend to be aggressive but keep this aggression under control particularly with persons they recognize as relatives. Knowledge of kinship is very important to humans. Altruism, or self-sacrificing, exists but more so for a relative than a nonrelative. In other words, the degree to which others share our genes influences our behavior toward them. This may be why small towns tend to have less crime than large cities.

Interestingly enough, various marriage habits around the world suggest a possible adaptation to the environment. Among African tribes, one man may

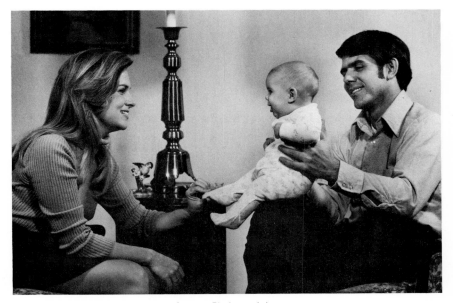

Figure 14.11 Human family group. (Source: Photograph by Harold M. Lambe.)

have several wives. This is reproductively advantageous to the male, but it is also advantageous to the woman since by this arrangement she has fewer children who are thereby assured a more nutritious diet. In Africa, sources of protein are scarce and protein deficiency diseases are a threat to continued existence.

Among the Bihari hillmen of India, brothers have one wife. The environment is hostile and it takes two men to provide the necessities for one family. The fact that the men are brothers means that they share genes in common and therefore they are actually helping each other look after common genes.

## Experiments in Human Reproductive Behavior

There have not been very many experiments in human social behavior, but the kibbutz in Israel is one such example. Here a real attempt was made to do away with the usual sex role differences. Men and women work alongside one another and the children are raised together in separate living quarters. Even so, there has developed a division of labor according to sex. The men do the more strenuous laboring jobs and the women do the customary "women's work"— washing clothes and preparing meals. Men tend to seek out positions of authority, whereas the women do not. Also, the women take more interest in their children, visiting them daily to establish a relationship with them that would otherwise not develop.

---

## Summary

Evolution occurs when organisms better suited to the environment survive, reproduce, and pass on their genotype to the next generation. Since these genotypes have been "selected," the process is called natural selection.

Sexual reproduction among diploid organisms presumably evolved from asexual reproduction among haploid organisms. A diploid genotype increases the chances of survival and is a source of genetic variation in addition to mutation. Sexual reproduction has been adapted to the land environment in plants and animals.

Evidence is presented to suggest that animal behavior is inherited and subject to the evolutionary process. Behavior increasing the chances of having offspring is favored. Baboon behavior is described to show that each sex has its own preferred behavioral patterns. Examples are given to show that human sexual behavior is suited to the environment. Thus, the possibility exists that human sexual behavior (including sexual roles) may be genetically determined, making it difficult for humans to assume roles other than those dictated by their genes. Sociobiologists believe that human male and female behavior has evolved to increase the chances of each sex passing their genes on to the next generation.

## Terms

adaptation

aggression

altruism

asexual reproduction

desiccation

dominance

evolution

genetic variation

natural selection

ovary

sexual reproduction

sociobiology

survival of the fittest

## Review

1. What are two drawbacks to asexual reproduction?
2. Define evolution, survival of the fittest, and adaptation.
3. What is the raw material for evolution? How does the sexual reproduction provide this?
4. How is reproduction in plants adapted to a land environment?
5. Compare the means of reproduction in frog and man to show that one is adapted to reproduction in water and the other to reproduction on land. Be sure to use the terms external and internal fertilization and external and internal development in your comparisons.
6. Give examples to show that behavior evolves and that reproductive behavior is adapted.
7. How might mammalian reproductive anatomy and physiology dictate the male and female behavior patterns?
8. Give an argument based on selection to show that the genes might control behavior appropriate to assuring their passage from one generation to another.
9. Discuss the tenets of sociobiology in relation to human behavior.
10. Discuss the possibility that "humans can overcome their basic biology."

# 15

# Biology of Sexual Behavior

Whatever control genes have on behavior, it is indirect control. Directly, the genes control the anatomy and physiology of the organism and only behavior allowed by the anatomy and physiology of the organism can occur. Figure 15.1 tells us that behavior suitable to the organism occurs as a response to environmental stimuli. Stimuli received by the sense receptors cause them to communicate with the central nervous system (CNS). The central nervous system interprets and integrates the incoming nerve impulses, thereafter directing the muscles to respond. The observed response is called the **behavior** of the organism. Often, the central nervous system must be in a state of readiness to respond. As will be discussed later, sexual readiness or motivation is believed to be dependent, at least in part, on hormonal levels.

Animals with simple nervous systems tend to respond only to certain stimuli automatically in a predetermined way, whereas animals with complex nervous systems tend to learn to respond to selected stimuli with behavior suited to the particular circumstances. All animals, including humans, show some behavior

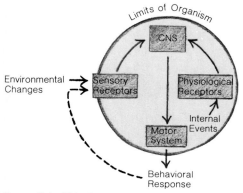

Figure 15.1   This diagram indicates that behavior is a response to a stimulus. The central nervous system (CNS) acts as the receiver and integrator of both external and internal stimuli. (After Nelson, *Fundamental Concepts of Biology*, John J. Wiley and Sons, 1974.)

of the first type, often called **innate** or **instinctive** behavior, but the higher animals have a larger component of learned behavior.

## External Stimuli

Humans have sense receptors that respond to external stimuli, such as odiferous stimuli, taste stimuli, visual stimuli, sound stimuli, and touch stimuli.

Lower mammalian animals are sexually stimulated by odors to a greater degree than humans. For example, female insects secrete chemicals called **pheromones** and male insects are so attracted by the smell that they will travel great distances to find a solitary female. Since the male insects respond automatically, synthetic pheromones can be used to capture male insects, eliminating the necessity to spray many acres of land with insecticides. Owners of dogs are also very much aware of the fact that their pets are stimulated by odors.

Experimentation is now being done to determine if humans are at all sexually stimulated by odorous chemicals produced by the opposite sex. Adult males are reported to secrete about twice as much of a chemical called exaltolide in their urine compared to females; while prepubertal children secrete none. Females are reported to have a vaginal chemical called copulin. Experimental results suggest that some apes and human subjects are capable of responding to these chemicals, while other subjects do not respond at all. In the same manner, only some subjects report that they are sexually stimulated by certain tastes.

Through the evolutionary process, apes and humans have become more dependent on visual stimuli than other types of stimuli. Males are reported to be more sensitive to visual sexual stimuli and it has been suggested that this is appropriate because an erection must occur before sexual intercourse is possible. However, these data are being challenged today since more women are willing to admit to being sexually aroused by visual and other stimuli.

Sounds such as music often set the appropriate mood for sexual excitement and sounds uttered during a sexual experience contribute to that experience, but, even so, sounds alone are not usually interpreted as sexually stimulating. The fantasizing that may accompany listening to music is classified as visual stimuli, since the subject is imagining different scenes in the mind's eye.

Along with sight and sounds, touch represents a major source of sexual excitement. Specific areas of the body become erotic zones when these areas have been touched under circumstances judged to be sexual. In other words, we learn to have various erotic zones. As mentioned in chapter 10, touch receptors accommodate to continuous stimuli so that they are no longer aroused. Thus, erogenous zones are better stimulated if they are stroked.

## Brain

Sense receptors communicate with the brain, which directs a response after these nerve impulses are received. Lower animals are programmed to respond in a certain manner so that actually the brain is simply a specialized relay station between sense receptors and the response. For example, male stickleback fish stake out a territory and build a nest; at this time the body becomes highly colored, including a red belly. Any male attempting to enter the territory is attacked as the owner repeatedly darts toward and nips the intruder. On the other hand, the owner entices a female to enter the territory by first darting toward her and then away in a so-called zig-zag dance (fig. 15.2). Finally, he leads her to the nest, where she deposits her eggs. How does the male stickleback recognize another male as opposed to a female? Experimentation has shown that males attack any model that has a red underside whether or not it resembles a fish (fig. 15.3). Therefore, the fish are believed to be programmed to respond automatically to sequential stimuli and are believed to carry out their reproductive behavior reflexively without the need for thought.

In humans, sense receptors also communicate with the brain (fig. 15.4), but in humans the brain is more apt to interpret the data and come to a decision

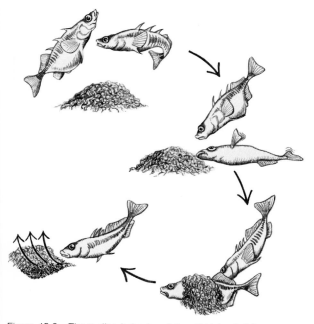

Figure 15.2   The mating behavior of the stickleback fish always has these components: the male entices the female to the nest, where he lies flat on his side; the female swims into the nest and lays her eggs when prodded by the male; finally, the male enters the nest to fertilize the eggs.

Evolution, Behavior, and Population

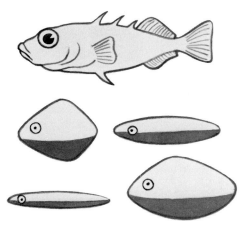

Figure 15.3   A red belly on a crude model stimulates females and males more than an exact replica of a fish without a red belly.

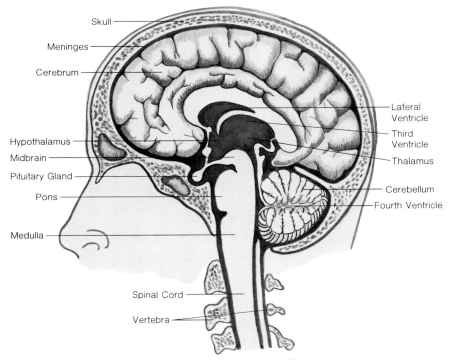

Figure 15.4   Human brain. (After Mader, *Inquiry into Life,* 2d edition.)

as to whether to respond and in what manner to respond. Some responses are automatic, but most are learned. Money and Ehrhardt state:

In the final analysis, all of a person's experience and behavior of falling in love and mating belongs to a program in the brain. Some parts of the program may have been phyletically laid down [by the evolutionary process]. Some may be the individualized product of prenatal hormonal history, and some the product of individual social history and learning. Whatever its origin, there is no behavior if it is not represented in the functioning of the brain.[1]

The human brain can be divided into three major sections: the hindbrain, the midbrain, and the forebrain. In the *hindbrain*, the **medulla oblongata** controls the internal organs and has centers for various reflex actions. Since the medulla is the most inferior portion of the brainstem, it functions as a pathway for sensory and motor impulses between the brain and the spinal cord, and vice versa. The reticular formation (fig. 15.5), a complex network of nerve cells and their processes, extends from the medulla to the thalamus. One portion of this, called the *ARAS* (**ascending reticular activating system**), is believed to

1. J. Money and A. Ehrhardt, *Man & Woman, Boy & Girl*
   (New York: New American Library, 1972), p. 245.

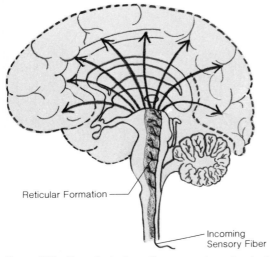

Reticular Formation

Incoming
Sensory Fiber

Figure 15.5 The reticular formation, a complex network of nerve cells, has one portion (represented by arrows) called the ascending reticular activation system (ARAS). (After Miller, M.A., Drakontides, A.B., and Leavell, L.C., *Anatomy and Physiology*, copyright © 1977 by Macmillan Publishing Co., Inc.)

alert higher centers to be prepared to receive information, including impulses that lead to sexual arousal.

The *forebrain* contains the hypothalamus, thalamus, and cerebrum. The **hypothalamus** is concerned with maintaining the body in a state of health and has centers for hunger, sleep, thirst, body temperature, water balance, and blood pressure. The pituitary gland is under the control of the hypothalamus, which along with the thalamus controls basic emotions and behavior.

The **thalamus** receives sensory impulses by way of the ARAS and passes this information along to the cerebrum. The thalamus plays the role of gatekeeper to the cerebrum, awakening it to only certain sensory input. The outer layer of the **cerebrum**, called the *cortex*, is highly convoluted and made up of lobes (fig. 15.6): the frontal lobes, the parietal lobes, the occipital lobe, and the temporal lobes. The *temporal lobes* are located at the sides of the head underneath the temples. Removal of these lobes produces hypersexual activity; therefore, it is possible that the temporal lobes ordinarily act to inhibit sexual behavior. The frontal lobes are associated with the most advanced human mental processes,

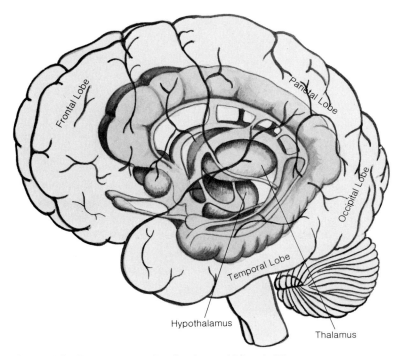

Figure 15.6   The human brain has four types of lobes. In this diagram the limbic system is the shaded area. (After Mader, *Inquiry into Life,* 2d edition.)

such as language, creativity, reasoning, and morals. It may be that the *frontal lobes* can direct the temporal lobes to keep sexual behavior under control.

Limbic System

The **limbic system** is an interconnected group of brain parts including portions of the frontal lobes, temporal lobes, thalamus, and hypothalamus, as well as pathways that connect all the parts together. Stimulation of different areas of the limbic system is believed to cause the subject to experience rage, pain, or pleasure. These **pleasure centers** are sometimes called self-stimulation centers because primarily animal subjects will repeatedly stimulate these centers if given the opportunity (fig. 15.7). The sensation is reported to be similar to that which accompanies orgasm. The actual feelings that accompany stimulation may be the province of the frontal lobes, while the manifested behavior such as sexual behavior may be determined by the types of impulses arriving at the limbic integrating center in the hypothalamus. Drugs that affect mood are known to particularly affect the ARAS and the limbic systems. Supposedly, drugs that stimulate the ARAS and limbic system and/or inhibit the thalamus would increase sexual enjoyment. So many drugs with diverse pharmacological activities have been reported to enhance the enjoyment of sex; however, it would appear that this effect may be due to the power of suggestion rather than to a neurological action of the drugs themselves.

## Hormones

Evidence suggests that hormones have three sexual effects in humans: (1) they affect not only the development of the sex organs but also the brain; (2) they promote the development of the secondary sex characteristics at puberty; and (3) they motivate sexual behavior.

As stated previously, persons with XY chromosomes develop into males with male genitalia when their tissues respond to androgens produced by the embryonic testes. There is a condition called the **androgen-insensitivity syndrome** in which the embryonic tissues are incapable of responding to androgens. XY individuals with this syndrome are born with immature testes and the genitalia of a female. Remarkably, they develop the secondary sex characteristics of females due to the estrogens produced by the adrenal cortex, and they prefer the gender identity and gender roles expected of females in our society.

In contrast, persons with XX chromosomes, whose tissues are capable of responding to androgens and who are accidentally exposed to androgens during development, are born with ovaries but also with varying degrees of malelike genitalia that can be surgically corrected.[2] Later, these females have behavioral

2. The mothers received a synthetic hormone, progestin, to prevent miscarriage. In rare cases, the hormone was metabolized to a form that had an unexpected androgen effect.

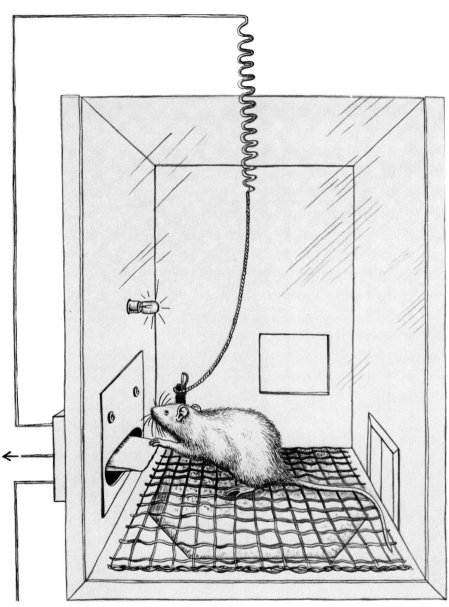

Figure 15.7   Animal subjects enjoy self-stimulation of pleasure
centers in order to experience the same sensations as sexual
arousal. (After Olds, J., ''Pleasure Centers in the Brain,''
*Scientific American*, Oct. 1956.)

characteristics described as "tomboyish" in that they like vigorous activity, are self-assertive, prefer functional clothing, and think of having a career before they think of romance and marriage. Human data of this type are limited, but the results have been substantiated by more extensive animal studies. These results have suggested to investigators that the presence or absence of androgens during some critical period of development does cause a *sexual dimorphism of the brain.* In other words, there may be a male brain as opposed to a female brain. The male-type brain develops if embryonic cells are capable of responding to the presence of androgens and the female-type brain develops if androgens are lacking or if the embryonic cells are incapable of responding to the presence of androgens (fig. 15.8).

Although **androgenized females** are inclined to delay marriage and motherhood, they still prefer heterosexual relationships. Thus far, it has been impossible to show that the presence of prenatal androgens in human females causes lesbianism. And certainly no relationship has been shown between postpubertal androgen or estrogen levels and homosexuality, bisexuality, or heterosexuality. The level of androgens in adults has been shown, however, to affect the sex drive; the higher the level of androgens in both sexes, the greater the sex drive. The adrenal cortex is the source of androgens in the female; and females are reported to be more receptive to sex whenever there is a greater proportion of androgens in relation to female hormones, such as just prior to menstruation and following menopause. Castrated males show a decline in sexual activity that is only alleviated once they are given testosterone therapy.

The increase in sex drive seen with androgens is believed to be due to their effect on the brain rather than their effect on the reproductive organs directly. This can be demonstrated in animals when a small hormone-containing pellet implanted in the hypothalamus increases sex drive. The amount of hormone in the pellet is too low to affect the reproductive organs directly; therefore, the effect must be directly on the brain.

In lower animals it can be seen that not only motivation but also subsequent sexual and reproductive activities are dependent on the presence of hormones. When male and female ring doves are separated one from the other, neither shows any tendency toward reproductive behavior. But when a pair are put together in a cage, the male begins courting by repeatedly bowing and cooing (fig. 15.9). Since castrated males do not do this, it can be reasoned that the hormone testosterone readies the male for this behavior. The sight of the male courting causes the pituitary gland in the female to release FSH and LH; these in turn cause her ovaries to produce eggs and release estrogen into the bloodstream. Now both male and female are ready to construct a nest, during which time copulation takes place. The hormone progesterone is believed to cause the birds to incubate the eggs and while they are incubating the eggs, the

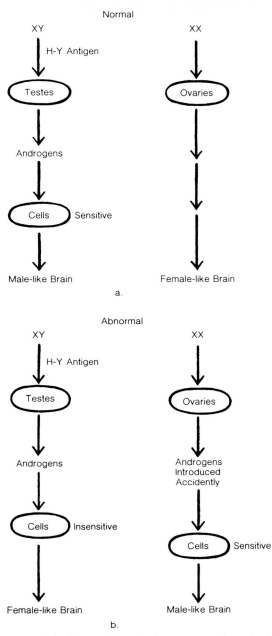

Figure 15.8   Diagram illustrating the sequence of events prior to the development of a male- or female-type brain.
(a) Normal sequence and (b) abnormal sequence.

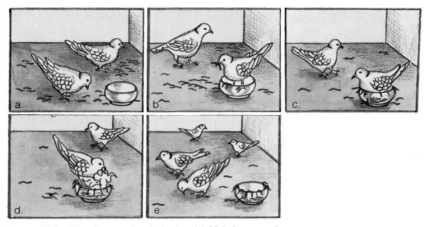

Figure 15.9 Ring dove mating behavior. (a) Male bows and coos; (b) nest building; (c) incubation of eggs; (d) baby birds are fed "crop milk"; and (e) cycle begins again.

hormone prolactin causes crop growth so that both parents are capable of feeding their young crop milk.

In humans, sequential reproductive activities may not be as dependent on hormonal levels because learning is so important to human behavior. In other words, in humans the presence or absence of hormones may cause motivation, but the actual activities are learned. This fact does not exclude the possibility that the inherent emotion associated with these activities might be the province of the genes. The fact that humans learn reproductive behavior can be substantiated by the fact that different cultures have their own preferred reproductive and sexual behavior.

It can be reasoned that the necessity to learn behavior means that isolated humans would be awkward in performing sexual behavior. Experimentation of this type is not possible in humans but has been done in monkeys. Males raised in isolation are clumsy and ineffective when given a chance to mate. In the previous chapter, we observed that human reproductive behavior might be controlled by genes, but in this chapter we have observed that the control must be indirect. Directly, sexual and reproductive behavior is controlled by the brain, which is motivated by hormonal levels but has learned to interpret certain stimuli as sexual stimuli, directing behavior that has been learned and yet can be varied to suit the particular circumstances.

## Summary

Behavior occurs as a response to environmental stimuli and is controlled by the brain. Odoriferous, taste, visual, sound, and touch stimuli can possibly sexually excite humans; the most important are believed to be visual and touch stimuli. Erogenous zones can vary from individual to individual.

The brain determines the behavioral response. In lower animals, the brain is most likely programmed genetically to direct the response automatically, but human behavior is largely learned. Human sexual behavior, including accompanying emotions, is most likely the province of the limbic integrating center of the brain.

Prenatally, hormones control the development of the sex organs and may even cause a sexual dimorphism of the brain. Hormones are also believed to affect the brain in adult life and to motivate human sexual behavior. The exact response humans make, however, is largely learned.

## Terms

androgen-insensitivity syndrome
cerebrum
frontal lobes
limbic system

medulla oblongata
reticular activating system
temporal lobes
thalamus

## Review

1. Discuss which sense data seem most important in humans in order to stimulate sexual activity.
2. Describe the reproductive behavior of stickleback fish. How do they respond to stimuli?
3. What is the ascending reticular activating system?
4. What parts of the brain make up the limbic system? Discuss the importance of the limbic system for sexual behavior.
5. Cite evidence for sexual dimorphism of the brain.
6. Has a connection been proven between level of hormones and homosexuality?
7. What effect do androgens have on sex drive in males? In females?
8. Describe the reproductive behavior of ring doves.
9. Contrast the control of human sexual behavior with ring dove behavior.

# 16            Human Population

The human growth curve is an exponential curve (fig. 16.1). In the beginning, growth of the population was relatively slow, but as greater numbers of reproducing individuals were added to the population, growth increased until the curve began to slope steeply upward. The slope of the curve at any one point shows how fast the population was increasing in size at that time. It is apparent from the position of 1980 on a growth curve of the human population that growth is now quite rapid.

At current rates, the world adds the equivalent of a medium-sized city every day (200,000) and the combined populations of the United Kingdom, Norway, Ireland, Iceland, Finland and Denmark every year. During the 1970s more than 700 million people will be added to the earth, more than in any previous decade and a figure larger than the total world population in 1700.[1]

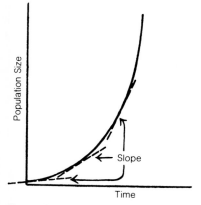

Figure 16.1   Exponential population growth. The slope of the curve at any one point shows how fast the population was increasing in size at that time. (Source: Adapted from *Biology: The Foundations* by Stephen L. Wolfe. © 1977 by Wadsworth Publishing Company, Inc., Belmont, California 94002. Reprinted by permission of the publisher.)

1. "Interchange," *Population Education Newsletter,* vol. 7, no. 2 (May 1978).

## World Growth Rate

The growth rate of a population is determined by subtracting the number of people that die from the number of individuals that are born per 100 persons per year. For example, if the death rate is 1.0 individuals while the birthrate is 3.0 individuals per 100 persons per year, then the growth rate for the year would be 2.0 individuals per 100 persons or 2 percent:

$$\text{G.R.} = \frac{3.0 - 1.0}{100} = 2\%$$

The growth rate for the world, which reached almost 2 percent, has declined slightly and yet the world population still increases in size because you must multiply the growth rate by the present population size in order to calculate the increase. For example, compare the annual increase of Population A, composed of 100 persons with a growth rate of 1.5 percent, to Population B, composed of 2,000 persons with a growth rate of 1.3 percent.

*Population A*

Population size = 100 persons
Growth rate = 1.5%
Annual increase = 1.5 persons

*Population B*

Population size = 2,000 persons
Growth rate = 1.3%
Annual increase = 26 persons

In other words, a small population with a large growth rate will not increase dramatically, whereas a large population with a modest growth rate is capable of increasing dramatically. The present world population is large—in 1650 there were about 500 million people in the world; in 1830 there were one billion; in 1930 there were 2 billion; in 1960 there were 3 billion; and in 1978 there were 4.2 billion. Since the world population is large, even a modest growth rate adds 73 million individuals to the population each year (fig. 16.2).

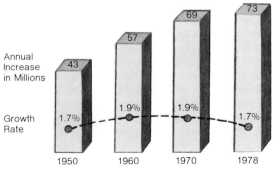

Figure 16.2   World population growth by decade. (Source: Courtesy of the Population Reference Bureau, Inc.)

*Doubling time.* With a growth rate of 1.7 percent, the world population is expected to double within 40 years. The doubling time for a population is calculated by dividing 70 (the demographic constant) by the growth rate:

$$D.T. = \frac{70}{1.7} \cong 40 \text{ years}$$

Many persons are now questioning if the world will be able to support the 8.6 billion persons expected by the year 2019 (1979 + 40). In other words, they ask the question, what is the carrying capacity of the earth?

Carrying Capacity

If the growth curve for nonhuman populations is examined, the population often tends to level off at a certain size. For example, figure 16.3 gives the actual data for the growth of a fruit fly population reared in a culture bottle. At the beginning, the fruit flies were becoming adjusted to their new environment and growth was slow. But then, since food and space were plentiful, they began to multiply rapidly. Notice that the curve begins to rise dramatically just as the human population curve does now. At this time, it may be said that the population is demonstrating its *biotic potential.* Biotic potential is the maximum growth rate under ideal conditions. Biotic potential is not usually demonstrated for long because of an opposing force called *environmental resistance.* Environmental resistance includes all the factors that cause early death of organisms and thus prevent the population from producing as many offspring as it might otherwise have done. As far as the fruit flies are concerned, we can speculate that environmental resistance included the limiting factors of food and space. Also, the waste given off by the fruit flies may have begun to contribute to keeping the population down.

The eventual size of any population represents a compromise between the biotic potential and the environmental resistance. This compromise occurs at the *carrying capacity* of the environment. The carrying capacity is the maximum population that the environment can support.

Experts have a difference of opinion as to the carrying capacity of the earth in regard to humans. Some authorities think the earth is potentially capable of supporting 50 to 100 billion people. Others think we already have more humans than the earth can support.

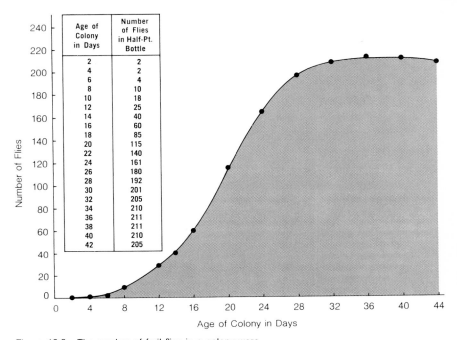

| Age of Colony in Days | Number of Flies in Half-Pt. Bottle |
|---|---|
| 2 | 2 |
| 4 | 2 |
| 6 | 4 |
| 8 | 10 |
| 10 | 18 |
| 12 | 25 |
| 14 | 40 |
| 16 | 60 |
| 18 | 85 |
| 20 | 115 |
| 22 | 140 |
| 24 | 161 |
| 26 | 180 |
| 28 | 192 |
| 30 | 201 |
| 32 | 205 |
| 34 | 210 |
| 36 | 211 |
| 38 | 211 |
| 40 | 210 |
| 42 | 205 |

Figure 16.3  The number of fruit flies in a colony were counted every other day, and when these numbers were plotted, a sigmoidal growth curve resulted (Courtesy of *Laboratory Studies in Biology: Observations and Their Implications* by Chester A. Lawson, Ralph W. Lewis, Mary Alice Burmester, and Garrett Hardin, W.H. Freeman and Co., San Francisco, Copyright ©, 1955).

### Developed and Underdeveloped Countries

While the growth rate and doubling time for the world is 1.7 percent and 40 years, respectively, each individual country can be studied separately (chart 16.1). Countries that tend to be nonindustrial are classified as underdeveloped and countries that are industrial are classified as developed. As the chart indicates, the underdeveloped countries are the ones that contribute most heavily to the world's growth rate. When the growth rate is analyzed for these countries, it is found that the death rate is on the decline while the birthrate is on the increase. This is causing the growth rate in these countries to increase, thus causing the population size to increase dramatically. It is estimated that in the year 2000 the population of the developed countries will be about 1.8 billion while the population of the underdeveloped countries will be about 5.2 billion (fig. 16.4).

## Chart 16.1

Current Overall Status of the Human Population and Its Major Subdivisions Is Given by These Numbers. The Figures Are for 1979, the Most Recent Year for Which Data and Estimates Are Available.

| Area | People (millions) | Crude Birth Rate (per 1,000 population per year) | Crude Death Rate (per 1,000 population per year) | Annual Rate of Population Growth (percent) |
|---|---|---|---|---|
| World | 4,321 | 28 | 11 | 1.7 |
| Developed countries | 1,173 | 16 | 9 | 0.7 |
| Underdeveloped countries | 3,148 | 33 | 12 | 2.1 |
| Africa | 457 | 46 | 17 | 2.9 |
| Asia | 2,498 | 29 | 11 | 1.8 |
| Latin America | 352 | 35 | 8 | 2.7 |
| U.S. | 220.3 | 15 | 9 | 0.6 |
| Oceania | 23 | 22 | 9 | 1.3 |
| Europe | 483 | 14 | 10 | 0.4 |
| U.S.S.R. | 264 | 18 | 10 | 0.8 |

Source: Population Reference Bureau, Inc.

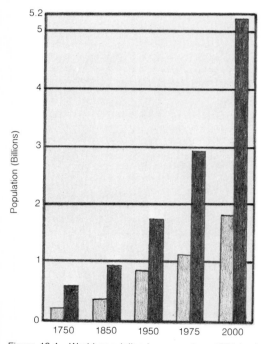

Figure 16.4   World population increase since 1750 is charted for developed countries (light) and underdeveloped countries (dark). Data for the year 2000 are based on a United Nations projection that assumes slowly ebbing growth rates. (From "The Populations of the Underdeveloped Countries" by Paul Demeny. Copyright © 1974 by Scientific American, Inc., All rights reserved.)

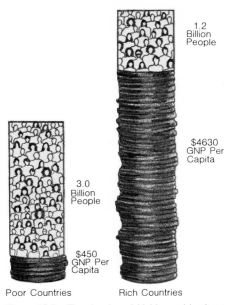

1.2
Billion
People

$4630
GNP Per
Capita

3.0
Billion
People

$450
GNP Per
Capita

Poor Countries      Rich Countries

Figure 16.5  The developed (rich) countries have a higher
gross national product per capita than the underdeveloped
(poor) countries (1978). (Source: Courtesy of the Population
Reference Bureau, Inc.)

At the current growth rates, most underdeveloped countries will double their population within 25 years and therefore will have to double their economic output within 25 years to keep their present standard of living. It's estimated that India needs 4 million new jobs each year in order to maintain the present standard of living, without even considering improving the standard of living.

Presently, the underdeveloped countries have a lower per capita gross national product (GNP) than do the developed countries (fig. 16.5). An increase in population without an increase in GNP causes a reduction in the per capita GNP of these countries. The income gap between the developed and underdeveloped countries (fig. 16.6) increased by more than 300 percent in 14 years because the latter countries failed to increase the GNP sufficiently. This gap might increase even greater in the next 14 years unless the population is stabilized. Therefore, governments in over 31 countries have instituted official policies to reduce population growth, and many of these countries are hoping to eventually achieve zero population growth (ZPG).

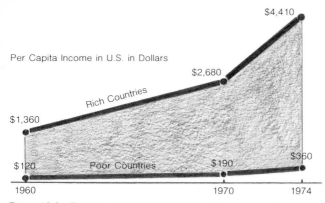

Figure 16.6 There is a widening gap between the per capita income of underdeveloped (poor) countries and developed (rich) countries. (Source: Courtesy of the Population Reference Bureau, Inc.)

## ZPG

Without exception, each country's growth rate is caused by the birthrate being higher than the death rate (chart 16.1). In every country, people are living longer than they used to; modern medicine and technology have increased the life span of all. Almost everyone would agree that the desirable way to bring about zero population growth is not to suddenly allow older people to die but to decrease the birthrate instead.

It is commonly believed that if each couple replaced only themselves (one couple having two children), then the population size would be stabilized at its present level. However, this is not the case because of the composition of most populations.

Figure 16.7 shows the composition of three different populations: one is that of an underdeveloped country (Mexico) and two are those of developed countries (United States and Sweden). The age profile for the population of Mexico exemplifies the shape of a young, expanding population because the proportion of persons in the prereproductive years (0–14) is higher than that of persons in the reproductive years (15–44), and the latter is higher than the postreproductive years (after 44). The rectangular-shaped profile of Sweden, on the other hand, is that of a stable population inasmuch as there are approximately the same number of persons in all three age categories. The United States falls somewhere between these two extremes and does not have an even proportion of persons in the three categories. This means that the United States will continue to have a population increase even if reproduction replacement were put into practice. *The World Almanac Book of Facts* states:

At present . . . there are nearly twice as many girls about to begin their childbearing years [in the U.S.] as there are women about to leave those years behind.

Evolution, Behavior, and Population

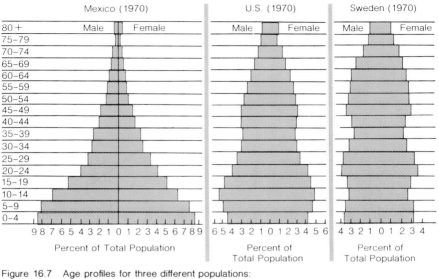

Figure 16.7   Age profiles for three different populations:
Mexico, United States, and Sweden. (From *The Human
Population,* by Ronald Freedman and Bernard Berelson.
Copyright © by Scientific American, Inc.).

While there are only 1,100,000 women who were 39 in 1973, there are 2,100,000
girls who were age 13. Even if the 13-year-olds only replace themselves, they
would produce nearly twice as many babies as the 39-year-olds. . . . That is,
70 years of low fertility [in the U.S.] are required to achieve population stability
at about 320 million people.[2]

Most of the underdeveloped nations have an age profile similar to that of
Mexico, while the developed nations are close to that of Sweden. However, since
two-thirds of the population is in the underdeveloped nations, this means that
the world as a whole has a youthful profile and that reproduction replacement
throughout the world would still produce many more people before the world's
population could begin to level off. This means that if the population is to level
off at its present level, on the average each couple should have less than two
children. While some couples could have two children, others should have one
or none.

## Results of Population Increase

Increased population has two general effects: (1) it increases the use of natural
resources and (2) it causes an increase in pollution.

2. From *The World Almanac and Book of Facts* (New York:
   Newspaper Enterprise Association, G.E. Delury, Exec. Ed.,
   1974). Used with permission.

*Natural resources.* Natural resources are classified as renewable and nonrenewable. Examples of renewable resources are food and water. Every time crops
are planted, more food is expected. Every time it rains, there is more water; the
water we use up is returned to us because water cycles (fig. 16.8). The definition
of renewable resources might cause us to think that there is no reason to worry
about the supply of these resources. But we are now very much aware of the
fact that the quantity of renewable resources cannot be expanded forever. Even
now we do not produce and equitably distribute enough food to feed all persons
adequately. And the possibility of producing and distributing enough to feed 8.4
billion seems doubtful. All the lands that we now know are capable of being
cultivated are under cultivation. Attempts have been made to bring other lands,
such as the tropics and deserts, under cultivation, but these attempts have as
yet not been successful. As a matter of fact, there are even indications that fresh
water is in limited supply. Water is now being diverted from less populated areas
to more populated areas. This suggests that there will not be an adequate water
supply if all areas become populated. Seawater can be desalted, but thus far
this has proven so expensive that it is not done extensively.

Nonrenewable resources are those that exist in limited amounts and once
they are used up they cannot be replaced. Many people do not realize that fuels
such as coal, oil, and natural gas fall into this category. These fuels are withdrawn
from stored quantities in the earth; once they have been depleted there will be

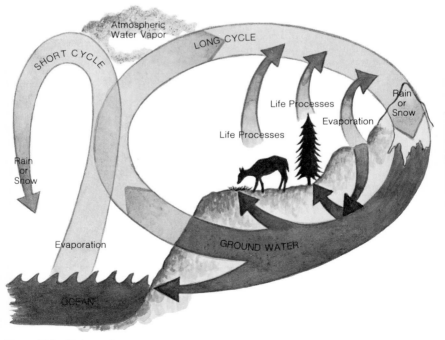

Figure 16.8   Water cycle.

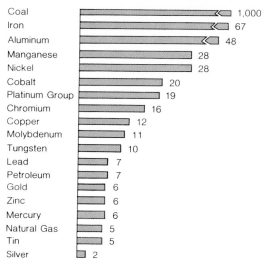

| | |
|---|---|
| Coal | 1,000 |
| Iron | 67 |
| Aluminum | 48 |
| Manganese | 28 |
| Nickel | 28 |
| Cobalt | 20 |
| Platinum Group | 19 |
| Chromium | 16 |
| Copper | 12 |
| Molybdenum | 11 |
| Tungsten | 10 |
| Lead | 7 |
| Petroleum | 7 |
| Gold | 6 |
| Zinc | 6 |
| Mercury | 6 |
| Natural Gas | 5 |
| Tin | 5 |
| Silver | 2 |

Figure 16.9    The number of years it may take to deplete world supply of each of these nonrenewable resources if the world population consumed at the United States rate. (Source: *Introduction to Environmental Science and Technology* by Gilbert M. Masters. Copyright © 1974 by John Wiley and Sons, Inc. Reprinted by permission of John Wiley and Sons, Inc.)

no more. Other resources of this type are given in figure 16.9, which shows the number of years it would take to deplete nonrenewable resources if the world consumed them at the same rate as the United States. The United States consumes natural resources at a rate higher than that of any other country in the world.

It is possible that technology can help ease the problem of possible shortages. Certainly, we can eventually devise means to make useable energy from renewable resources. For example, oil and coallike pellets can be made from garbage, but it may take time to perfect the process. Also with time, solar energy can replace fossil fuels for certain purposes, such as heating our homes. Some question, however, that there would be enough time to develop these methods to meet the energy needs if the world population doubles within 40 years.

While the possibility exists that technology can solve certain shortage problems, we are now very much aware that advanced technology goes hand in hand with pollution. The largest polluter of air is not factories but the automobile (chart 16.2). The more people there are, the more cars that will be on the road and the greater the pollution. Even with stricter emission standards today, the amount of pollution due to the automobile stays the same because of the increased numbers of automobiles.

Technology can increase the amount of food by developing new breeds of plants that produce a higher yield than the parent plants. But such plants

**Chart 16.2** Air pollution contains five major components: CO (carbon monoxide), HC (hydrocarbons), $NO_x$ (nitrogen oxides), particulates (solid matter), $SO_x$ (sulfur oxides). Transportation contributes most to air pollution. (From *Introduction to Environmental Science and Technology* by Gilbert M. Masters. Copyright © 1974 by John Wiley and Sons, Inc. Reprinted by permission of John Wiley and Sons, Inc.)

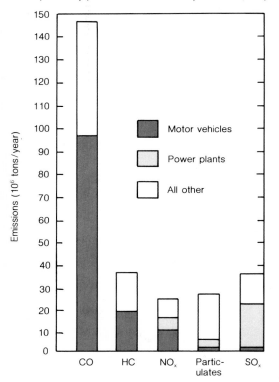

require increased amounts of fertilizer and frequent spraying with pesticides. Both of these procedures eventually cause pollution.

Aside from these considerations, humans, as biological creatures, produce pollution. Most of our rivers today are open sewers, carrying not only waste from factories but also human waste. It is against the law in most areas to dump raw sewage into rivers, but the process still continues in areas where no laws exist or where enforcement is lacking. Every city and town should be putting considerable funds into constructing sewage treatment plants. In a primary treatment plant, solids, grease, and scum are removed; in a secondary treatment plant (fig. 16.10), any remaining organic matter is dissolved by bacterial action; in a tertiary treatment plant, nutrient molecules are removed to prevent overgrowth of the water's natural inhabitants, such as algae. The cost for primary and secondary treatment plants is given in figure 16.11. It is estimated that a tertiary plant costs twice that of a secondary one.

Evolution, Behavior, and Population

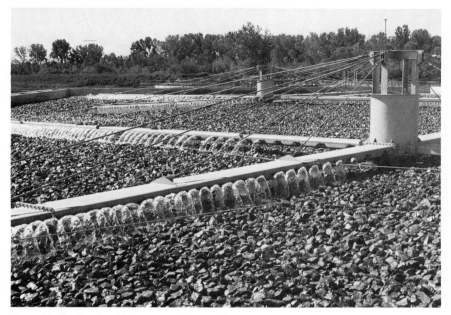

Figure 16.10   The Des Moines, Iowa, Sewage Treatment
Plant. The sewage is treated through a series of filters,
clarifiers, grease removal tanks, and sludge digesters before
the water is considered suitable for return to the Des Moines
River. (Source: EPA, Office of Public Affairs.)

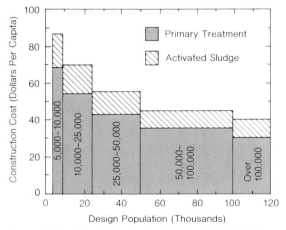

Figure 16.11   Construction cost of primary and secondary
(activated sludge) treatment plants per capita varies according
to the size of the town or city. (From *Introduction to
Environmental Science and Technology* by Gilbert M. Masters.
Copyright © 1974 by John Wiley and Sons, Inc. Reprinted by
permission of John Wiley and Sons, Inc.)

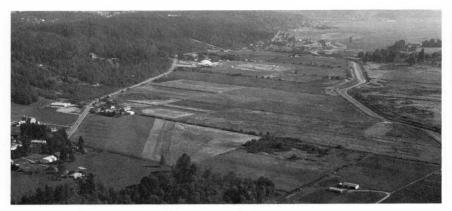

Figure 16.12    Housing development. (Source: U.S. Dept. of
Agriculture.)

Another type of pollution that we are all concerned about is the loss of open spaces. The popular song suggesting that we may eventually pay "a dollar and a half" to see a tree asks us to see the value of natural settings that have not been spoiled by construction (fig. 16.12). Humans tend to replace natural settings with artificial ones; our love of open places tells us that this is not an altogether desirable occurrence. Some persons have suggested that if it gets too crowded on this planet, people could be transported to other planets. Two authorities have estimated that at the current rate of population increase, the United States would have to spend 20 times its gross national product annually to export the people who are being added to its population every year.[3] Clearly, then, this is not a feasible suggestion. It seems much more reasonable to realize that all of us must find suitable living space on the outside crust of a small sphere (fig. 16.13) and there is no more room than this.

## Summary

At the present time, the population of the world is undergoing exponential growth and therefore even though the annual growth rate has declined slightly the world population still continues to increase dramatically. Most of this increase will occur in the underdeveloped countries rather than the developed ones. The underdeveloped countries tend to have a pyramid-shaped age profile indicating that a very large number of individuals are young and will be entering the reproductive years. Therefore, replacement reproduction would not immediately bring about zero population growth.

3. I.M. Lerner and W.J. Libby, *Hereditary, Evolution and Society* (San Francisco: W.H. Freeman, 1976), p. 264.

Evolution, Behavior, and Population

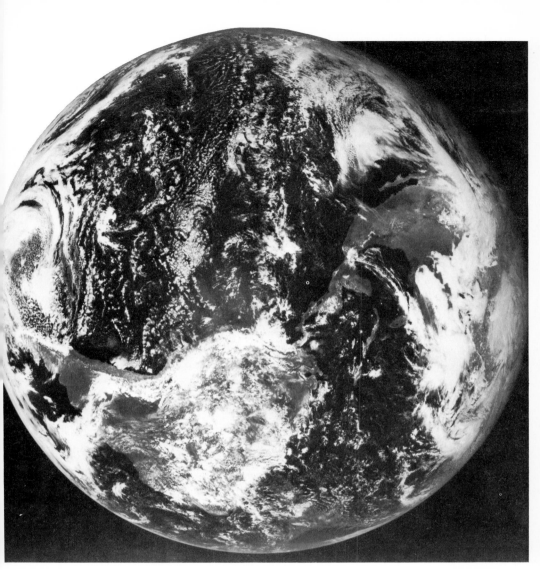

Figure 16.13 All of us must find room on the outer crust of a planet of finite size. (Courtesy of National Aeronautics and Space Administration.)

It is a serious question as to whether the earth is already overpopulated with people. We are incapable of feeding the masses; water, fossil fuels, and other resources are also in short supply. While many believe that technology will be able to overcome all these difficulties, we now know that technology itself can create ecological problems. Since the earth has a finite carrying capacity it might be well to realize that the human population cannot continue to increase indefinitely.

## Terms

biotic potential
carrying capacity
developed and underdeveloped
    countries
doubling time
environmental resistance

growth rate
natural resources (renewable and
    nonrenewable)
tertiary sewage treatment plants
zero population growth

## Review

1. What is the formula for growth rate? If the birthrate is 0.9 percent and the death rate is 0.2 percent for a certain population, what would be the growth rate?
2. What is the formula for doubling time? What is the doubling time for the population mentioned in review question number 1?
3. Explain why a smaller population rather than a large population can tolerate a high growth rate and a short doubling time.
4. Draw a growth curve that levels off to a stable population. Where on the curve would you indicate biotic potential, environmental resistance, carrying capacity?
5. How do underdeveloped countries differ from developed countries in terms of industrialization, growth rates, doubling time?
6. What is ZPG? Why can't it be achieved now in the U.S. by each couple having two children?
7. What are the two general effects of increased population? Give examples of both.
8. Outline a long-term program by which each city and town could help clean up the rivers.
9. Argue the pros and cons of having technology solve shortage problems created by increased consumption.

## Further Readings for Part 3

Barash, D.P. 1977. *Sociobiology and Behavior.* New York: Elsevier North-Holland, Inc.

Dawkins, R. 1976. *The Selfish Gene.* New York: Oxford University Press.

*Ecology, Evolution and Population Biology.* 1974. Readings from *Scientific American.* San Francisco: W.H. Freeman & Co.

Ehrlich, P.R., et al. 1973. *Human Ecology: Problems and Solutions.* San Francisco: W.H. Freeman & Co.

Gardner, R. 1972. *The Baboon.* New York: The Macmillan Company.

Miller, G.T., Jr. 1979. *Living in the Environment: Concepts, Problems and Alternatives.* 2nd ed. Belmont, Calif.: Wadsworth Publishing Co.

Money, J., and Ehrhardt, A.A. 1972. *Man and Woman, Boy and Girl.* Baltimore: Johns Hopkins University Press.

Olds, J. 1956. Pleasure centers in the brain. *Scientific American* 195 (4):105–116.

Savage, J.M. 1977. *Evolution.* 3rd ed. New York: Holt, Rinehart and Winston.

*Scientific American.* 1974. 231(3), entire issue devoted to human population.

Volpe, E. 1977. *Understanding Evolution.* Dubuque, Iowa: Wm. C. Brown Company Publishers.

Westoff, C.F. 1978. Marriage and fertility in the developed countries. *Scientific American* 239(6):51.

# Epilogue

Sexual reproduction in humans facilitates the passage of genes from one generation to another. At fertilization two gametes join and with this union a new life begins. The biological heritage that parents give their children is contained within the two gametes. The quality of the genes will influence the eventual health and well-being of the offspring. Fortunately, it is possible for parents to determine in some instances if they have a faulty gene and therefore it is possible for them to prevent the passage of this gene or prevent the illness that will come due to the passage of the gene. Much of modern genetic research is aimed at curing and/or alleviating human genetic diseases.

Physiological functions of human beings are carried out by various organ systems. The reproductive system contains those organs that produce, store, transfer or receive gametes. The sex drive in humans encompasses not only biological but also psychological fulfillment. The manner in which these drives are fulfilled is largely learned by a constant interaction between the human organism and the environment. With the conception, birth, and growth of a new individual the procreative urge has been brought to fruition, but since the sex drive is not purely dependent upon this urge, conception can be prevented by the use of birth control. The possibility of venereal disease can also be prevented in many instances by sound health practices.

Do humans basically engage in sex because they are driven to do so by their genetic inheritance? Is reproductive behavior, including gender roles, a product of the evolutionary process? No matter whether the answer to these questions is affirmative or negative, behavior is still dependent on the nervous system. If genes do control behavior, they must first direct the development of a brain that will have the human organism strive to do their bidding. There is some evidence to suggest that chromosomal inheritance determines either a male or female-type brain. Sexual behavior, which seems to have both inherited and learned aspects, has resulted in a very large human population. Human beings act as if they wish to fulfill their biotic potential, and in this regard, they resemble all other species on earth. However, humans are unlike other species because of their great capacity to learn. Humans are able to work to increase the carrying capacity of the earth, and they can also purposefully keep the population in check. Social efforts have been and most likely will be directed toward both these goals.

# Appendix

## A.
## Genetic
## Diseases

We now know that a number of diseases in humans are genetically inherited. Some of the more frequently inherited conditions are listed below.

### Dominant

Currently, some 1,489 dominantly inherited disorders have been catalogued. Examples include:

- achondroplasia—a form of dwarfism
- chronic simple glaucoma (some forms)—a major cause of blindness if untreated
- Huntington's disease—progressive nervous system degeneration
- hypercholesterolemia—high blood cholesterol levels, propensity to heart disease
- polydactyly—extra fingers or toes

### Recessive

Among 1,117 recessively inherited disorders catalogued are:

- cystic fibrosis—disorder affecting function of mucus and sweat glands
- galactosemia—inability to metabolize milk sugar
- phenylketonuria—essential liver enzyme deficiency
- sickle cell disease—blood disorder primarily affecting blacks
- thalassemia—blood disorder primarily affecting persons of Mediterranean ancestry

### Sex-linked

Among 205 catalogued disorders transmitted by a gene or genes on the X chromosome are:

- agammaglobulinemia—lack of immunity to infections
- color blindness—inability to distinguish certain colors
- hemophilia—defect in blood-clotting mechanisms
- muscular dystrophy (some forms)—progressive wasting of muscles
- spinal ataxia (some forms)—spinal cord degeneration

### Multiple genes

The number of defects due to multifactorial inheritance is unknown. Some that are thought to be multifactorial are:

- cleft lip and/or palate
- clubfoot
- congenital dislocation of the hip
- spina bifida—open spine
- hydrocephalus (with spina bifida)—water on the brain
- pyloric stenosis—narrowed or obstructed opening from stomach into small intestine

Data from the National Foundation/March of Dimes

# B.
## Sources of Information

American Association of Marriage and Family Counselors, 225 Yale Ave., Claremont, Cal. 91711

American Association of Sex Educators, Counselors, and Therapists, 5010 Wisconsin Ave., N.W., Washington, D.C. 20016

American Citizens Concerned for Life, 6127 Excelsior Blvd., Minneapolis, Minn. 55416

American Fertility Society, 1608 13th Ave., S., Suite 101, Birmingham, Ala. 35205

American Institute of Family Relationships, 5287 Sunset Blvd., Los Angeles, Cal. 90027

American Social Health Association, 260 Sheridan Ave., Suite 307, Palo Alto, Cal. 94306

Association for Voluntary Sterilization, Inc., 708 Third Ave., New York, N.Y. 10017

Barren Foundation, 6 E. Monroe Street, Chicago, Ill. 60603

E.C. Brown Foundation, 710 S.W. Second Ave., Portland, Ore., 97204

Choice, 1501 Cherry St., Philadelphia, Pa. 19102

Institute for Sex Research, Inc., Indiana University, Bloomington, Ind. 47401

Janus Information Facility Gender Clinic, 415 Texas Ave, 2nd Floor Unit D (University of Texas, Medical Branch), Galveston, Tex. 77550

Maternity Center Association, 48 East 92nd St., New York, N.Y. 10028

Mattachine Society of New York, 59 Christopher St., New York, N.Y. 10014

National Family Planning Council, 7060 Hollywood Blvd., Suite 414, Los Angeles, Cal. 90028

National Sex Forum, 1523 Franklin St., San Francisco, Cal. 94109

Planned Parenthood—World Population, 810 Seventh Ave., New York, N.Y. 10019

Population Council, One Dag Hammarskjold Plaza, New York, N.Y. 20017

Population Reference Bureau, 1755 Massachusetts Ave., N.W., Washington, D.C. 20036

Scientists for Life, 1908 Washington Ave., Fredericksburg, Va. 22401

Sex Information and Education Council of the U.S., 84 Fifth Ave., Suite 407, New York, N.Y. 10011

Society for Scientific Study of Sex, 12 East 41st St., Suite 1104, New York, N.Y. 10017

World Population Society, 1337 Connecticut Ave., N.W., Suite 200, Washington, D.C. 20036

Zero Population Growth, 1346 Connecticut Ave., N.W., Washington, D.C. 20036

# C.
## Journals

### American Journal of Obstetrics and Gynecology

American Gynecological Society
C.V. Mosby Co.
11830 Westline Industrial Drive
St. Louis, Mo 63141

### Archives of Andrology

Elsevier North Holland, Inc.
52 Vanderbilt Avenue
New York, N.Y. 10017

### Archives of Sexual Behavior

Plenum Publishing Corp.
227 W. 17th Street
New York, N.Y. 10011

### Biology of Reproduction

The Society for the Study of
Reproduction
113 North Neil Street
Champaign, Il 61820

### Child and Family

National Commission on Human Life,
Reproduction, and Rhythm
Box 508
Oak Park, Il 60303

### Contraception

Geron-X, Inc.
Box 1108
Los Altos, California 94022

### Early Human Development

Elsevier North Holland, Inc.
52 Vanderbilt Avenue
New York, N.Y. 10017

### Fertility and Sterility

American Fertility Society
1608 13th Avenue South
Birmingham, Alabama 35205

### Journal of Marriage and the Family

National Council on Family Relations
1219 University Avenue Southeast
Minneapolis, Mn 55414

### Journal of Population

American Psychological Association
Human Sciences Press
72 Fifth Avenue
New York, N.Y. 10011

### Journal of Nurse-midwifery

American College of Nurse-midwifery
Elsevier North Holland, Inc.
52 Vanderbilt Avenue
New York, N.Y. 10017

### Journal of Reproductive Immunology

Elsevier North Holland Inc.
52 Vanderbilt Avenue
New York, N.Y. 10017

### Journal of Sex and Marital Therapy

Human Sciences Press
72 Fifth Avenue
New York, N.Y. 10011

### Journal of Sex Research

Society for the Scientific Study of Sex
12 East 41st Street, Suite 1104
New York, N.Y. 10017

### Obstetrical and Gynecological Survey

Williams and Wilkins Co.
428 E. Preston Street
Baltimore, Maryland 21202

### Obstetrics and Gynecology

American College of Obstetricians and
Gynecologists
Elsevier North Holland, Inc.
52 Vanderbilt Avenue
New York, N.Y. 10017

### Sex Roles

Plenum Publishing Corporation
227 W. 17th Street
New York, N.Y. 10011

### Sexuality and Disability

Human Sciences Press
72 Fifth Avenue
New York, N.Y. 10011

### Sexually Transmitted Diseases

J.B. Lippincott Co.
East Washington Square
Philadelphia, Pa 19105

### Siecus Report

Sex Information and Education Council of
the U.S.
84 Fifth Avenue
New York, N.Y. 10011

# Glossary

**acrosome**
A cap over the sperm head that contains enzymes believed to assist the process of fertilization.

**adaptation**
The fitness of an organism for its environment, including the process by which it becomes fit, in order that it may survive and reproduce.

**adrenal glands**
Endocrine glands that lie atop the kidneys.

**afterbirth**
The placenta and extraembryonic membranes that are expelled following the birth of a baby.

**altruism**
Self-sacrifice.

**amino acid**
A subunit of a protein.

**amniocentesis**
The removal of a small amount of amniotic fluid to examine the chromosomes and the enzymatic potential of fetal cells.

**amnion**
The extraembryonic membrane containing the amnionic fluid that bathes the embryo and fetus.

**androgen-insensitivity syndrome**
Persons with XY chromosomes and testes who have the genitals and secondary sex characteristics of females because their tissues are incapable of responding to androgens.

**androgens**
Male sex hormones of which testosterone is the most potent.

**anther**
That portion of the stamen (male part of flower) that produces pollen.

**antibodies**
Chemicals made by an individual to react with and thereby combat antigens.

**antigens**
A foreign substance that causes the individual to form antibodies.

**areola**
A colored ring of tissue surrounding the nipple of the breast.

**arterial duct**
A fetal blood vessel that takes blood from the pulmonary trunk to the aorta so that blood from the right side of the heart bypasses the lungs.

**asexual reproduction**
Reproduction that requires only one parent and does not involve gametes.

**autosomal dominant**
A dominant gene that is carried on an autosomal chromosome, which may be present singularly for characteristic to be seen phenotypically.

**autosomal recessive**
A recessive gene that is carried on an autosomal chromosome, which must be present in duplicate for the characteristic to be seen phenotypically.

**autosome**
Any chromosome other than sex chromosomes. In humans there are 22 pairs of autosomes.

**bases**
A subunit of a nucleotide. In DNA nucleotides the bases are adenine, thymine, guanine, and cytosine. In RNA nucleotides the bases are adenine, uracil, guanine, and cytosine.

**bestiality**
Human sexual contact with animals.

**biochemical genetics**
DNA structure and function.

**biotic potential**
The reproductive ability of a population when environmental conditions are ideal.

**bisexual**
A person who has sex with persons of both genders.

**bubo**
Inflammatory swelling of a lymph node.

**bulbourethral glands**
See Cowper's glands.

**capacitation**
A maturation process that usually occurs within the vagina, enabling sperm to fertilize an egg.

**carrier**
A hybrid individual that appears normal, but who carries a recessive gene for genetic disease.

**carrying capacity**
The maximum number of organisms that an environment can support.

**cell**
The smallest unit of life.

**cerebrum**
The main portion of the vertebrate brain that is responsible for consciousness.

**chance**
The probability of inheriting a particular characteristic.

**chancre**
A small papule that becomes an open sore where an organism invaded the body.

**chloasma**
Pigmented patches of skin on the face and neck that develop during pregnancy, menstruation, or when taking the birth control pill.

**chorion**
The extraembryonic membrane that lies outside the amnion and becomes part of the placenta.

**chromatids**
The two identical parts of a duplicated chromosome.

**chromosomes**
Rod-shaped bodies in the nucleus, particularly visible during cell division, which contain the genes.

**circumcision**
Removal of the foreskin from the penis.

**climacteric**
A period of time in men, characterized by physiological and emotional disturbances.

**clitoris**
A slightly erectile organ of females that is homologous to the penis.

**cloning**
Development of a normal, sexually reproducing organism with the same genotype as the donor; a diploid nucleus inserted into an enucleated egg.

**coitus**
Sexual intercourse.

**coitus interruptus**
An abrupt withdrawal of the penis to prevent sperm from entering the vagina; a birth control measure.

**complementary base pairing**
The attraction of certain nucleotide bases to one another. In DNA, adenine always pairs with thymine and guanine always pairs with cytosine, and vice versa. If RNA nucleotides pair with DNA nucleotide, adenine always pairs with uracil and guanine always pairs with cytosine, and vice versa.

**condom**
A sheath that fits over the erect penis, preventing the sperm from entering the vagina; a birth control device.

**congenital**
Any condition present at birth.

**congenital syphilis**
Syphilis contracted during embryonic or fetal development.

**Cooley's anemia**
A genetic disease characterized by weak red cells.

**copulation**
Sexual intercourse.

**corpora cavernosa**
Two longitudinal masses of erectile tissue in the penis that lie above the urethra.

**corpus luteum**
A body, yellow in color, which forms in the ovary from a follicle that has discharged its egg. It secretes progesterone.

**corpus spongiosum**
Longitudinal mass of erectile tissue in the penis that surrounds the urethra.

**Cowper's glands**
Glands that lie on either side of the urethra, which secrete fluids that are a part of seminal fluid.

**Cri du Chat**
A syndrome in children caused by a shortened number 5 chromosome. Characterized by a small head, malformations of the head and body, mental defectiveness, and a cry similar to a kitten's meow.

**cunnilingus**
Oral stimulation of the female genitalia, especially the clitoris.

**curettage**
Scraping the inside of a cavity, such as the uterus, by means of a curette.

**curette**
A surgical instrument, shaped like a spoon, used to scrape the inside of cavities.

**cytoplasm**
The fluid portion of the cell located outside the nucleus.

**D & C**
Dilation and curettage—a surgical operation that involves dilation of the cervix and insertion of a curette to scrape the uterus clean of its contents.

**DES**
Diethylstilbestrol, a synthetic estrogen that is sometimes used as a morning-after birth control pill.

**desiccation**
Drying out due to lack of water.

**detumescence**
The return of an erect penis to its normal, flaccid state.

**developed countries**
Industrialized countries with a high Gross National Product (GNP) per capita.

**diaphragm**
A cup-shaped birth control device that fits over the cervix.

**dimorphic**
Species members that exist in two different forms. For example, in humans, males and females have different appearances.

**diploid number**
The 2N number of chromosomes; the complete or total number; twice the number of chromosomes found in gametes.

**DNA**
Deoxyribonucleic acid, the hereditary material.

**dominance**
In behavior, the presence of a pecking order by which some animals exert control over other animals.

**double helix**
A double spiral used to describe the three-dimensional shape of DNA.

**doubling time**
The number of years it takes for a population to double in size.

**douche**
A cleansing of the vagina with a solution.

**Down's syndrome**
A syndrome most often caused by the individual inheriting three number 21 chromosomes. Characterized by eyes that appear Oriental and mental retardation.

**ductus deferentia (s. ductus deferens)**
Ducts that lie between the epididymides and the urethra where the sperm are stored before entering the urethra during emission.

**duplication**
The process by which DNA makes a copy of itself.

**E. coli**
A bacterium that normally lives within the human gut and is often cultivated in the laboratory.

**ectopic pregnancy**
An implantation of the zygote in a location other than the uterus.

**effacement**
The dilation of the cervix during parturition.

**ejaculation**
The release of semen from an erect penis; transport of semen from the body.

**embryo**
That stage of development from fertilization to the end of the second month.

**emission**
Movement of sperm from the ductus deferentia to the urethra.

**endocrine glands**
Glands of internal secretion that produce hormones.

**endometrium**
The lining of the uterus.

**environmental resistance**
Environmental factors that prevent a population from achieving its biotic potential.

**enzymes**
Protein molecules that speed up a chemical reaction in cells.

**epididymides (s. epididymis)**
Coiled tubules where the sperm mature after being produced in the seminiferous tubules and before entering the ductus deferentia.

**episotomy**
Incision of the vaginal opening to facilitate birth.

**erection**
Process by which the penis becomes firm and erect; word that refers to the penis being erect, or nonflaccid.

**erogenous zone**
Any portion of the body that causes sexual excitement when touched.

**erythroblastosis**
Rh factor disease caused by an Rh— mother forming antibodies against the Rh+ red cells of the fetus.

**estrogen**
One type of female sex hormone, the other being progesterone.

**evolution**
Genetic changes that occur in populations of organisms with the passage of time, resulting in increasing adaptation of the organism to the prevailing environment.

**exhibitionist**
A public display of the genitals for the purpose of attracting sexual interest.

**expulsion**
The second phase of ejaculation when the semen is released from the penis.

**extraembryonic membranes**
Membranes that envelop the embryo and later the fetus.

**fallopian tubes**
Oviducts.

**feedback control**
A system of regulation by which the increase in a product leads to a decrease in its production and vice versa.

**fellatio**
Oral stimulation of the penis.

**fertilization**
Union of a sperm with an egg.

**fetishism**
The condition of being sexually stimulated by an object or part of the body generally considered inappropriate for sexual purposes.

**fetus**
That stage of development from the end of the second month to birth.

**follicle**
*See* ovarian follicle.

**follicular phase**
That part of the ovarian cycle when a follicle is maturing, prior to ovulation.

**foreplay**
Activities that cause sexual arousal; sexual activities that precede sexual intercourse.

**frontal lobes**
Anterior lobes of the cerebrum that are believed to be responsible for unique human faculties such as language, creativity, and morals.

**gametes**
Reproductive cells, e.g., sperm and egg.

**gametogenesis**
Production of gametes by the process of meiosis and maturation.

**gender identity**
The identification of self as male or female.

**gender role**
Behavior appropriate to gender identity.

**gene**
A unit of heredity located on a chromosome and composed of DNA.

**genetic disease**
A medical condition that is inherited genetically.

**genetic engineering**
Any human modification of genetic systems.

**genetic variation**
Genotype changes such as those due to mutation and recombination.

**genotype**
The genetic makeup of an individual.

**germinal mutation**
A mutation that occurs during the production of sperm and eggs.

**gerontophilia**
The desire to have sexual contact with old people.

**gonadotropic hormones**
Hormones produced by the anterior pituitary that stimulate the gonads to produce gametes and hormones.

**gonad**
An organ that produces sex cells; ovary and testis.

***Gonorrhea gonococcus***
The bacterium that causes gonorrhea infection.

**graffian follicle**
An ovarian follicle characterized by a cavity with the egg to one side.

**growth rate**
Population growth that is calculated by subtracting the annual death rate from the annual birth rate.

**gumma**
A soft, gummy tumor occurring in tertiary syphilis.

**haploid number**
The N number of chromosomes; half the diploid number; the number characteristic of gametes, which contain only one set of chromosomes.

**hemophilia**
A sex-linked genetic disease characterized by excessive bleeding because the blood does not clot.

**HCGTH**
Human chorionic gonadotropic hormone, a hormone produced by the placenta.

**heterosexual**
A person who prefers to have a sexual relationship with a person of the opposite sex.

**homosexual**
A person who prefers to have a sexual relationship with a person of the same sex.

**hormone**
A chemical produced by one set of cells in the body that affects a different set of cells.

**Huntington's chorea**
A genetic disease that leads to neurological impairment.

**Hutchinson's teeth**
A type of teeth found in persons who had congenital syphilis.

**H-Y antigen**
A protein that causes the embryonic gonads to develop into testes.

**hybrid**
A genotype having one dominant and one recessive gene for a characteristic, such as Ee. Phenotypically, shows the dominant characteristic.

**hymen**
A thin, stretchable membrane partially covering the vaginal opening.

**hypothalamus**
A part of the brain that controls the pituitary gland and is involved in various emotional states.

**immunity**
The ability to produce antibodies against a particular disease.

## implantation
A zygote embedding itself in the uterine lining.

## impotency
The inability to achieve or sustain an erection.

## interstitial cells
Cells that lie between the seminiferous tubules in the testes and produce androgens.

## intrauterine device (IUD)
A small coil or loop, usually made of plastic, that is placed in the uterus to prevent pregnancy.

## in vitro
Within a glass; observable in a test tube.

## in vivo
Within a living body.

## karyotype
A display of an individual's chromosomes arranged by pairs to show the number, size, and shape of the chromosomes.

## Klinefelter's syndrome
A condition characterized by the sex chromosomes XXY, usually showing some feminization of features.

## labia majora
Two large folds of skin that constitute the outer lips of the vulva; homologous to scrotum of male.

## labia minora
Two small folds lying between the labia majora.

## labium (pl. labia)
*See* labia majora and labia minora.

## labor
A period of cervical contractions prior to birth.

## ladder structure
Double-stranded DNA excluding the twisting that creates a spiral.

## laparoscopy
Examination of the abdominal cavity by means of a telescopic-type instrument with a cold light source.

## Lesch Nyhan syndrome
A sex-linked genetic condition characterized by self-mutilation.

## lesbian
A woman who prefers to have a sexual relationship with another woman.

## limbic system
An interconnected group of parts of the forebrain that is believed to be important in regulating the emotions.

## luteal phase
That part of an ovarian cycle after ovulation when the corpus luteum is maturing and then degenerating.

## masochist
A person who is sexually aroused when physically mistreated by a sexual partner.

## masturbation
Sexual pleasure, especially orgasm, obtained by stimulation, usually by means of manual manipulation.

## medulla oblongata
The lowest portion of the brain that is concerned with the control of internal organs.

## meiosis
Cell division in which the four daughter cells have half the number and one of each kind of chromosomes as the original mother cell.

## menarche
First occurrence of the menstrual discharge.

## menopause
Cessation of the menstrual cycle.

## menses
Degeneration of the uterine lining causing a discharge; also called menstruation.

## menstrual cycle
Usually a 28-day cycle during which the uterine lining first thickens, becomes secretory, and then degenerates.

## metabolic disease
A medical condition that is caused by the inheritance of a faulty gene that codes for a nonfunctioning enzyme.

## microorganisms
Small organisms that must be seen with a microscope.

## mitosis
Cell division in which the two daughter cells have the same number and kind of chromosomes as the mother cell.

## mongolism
See Down's syndrome.

## mons pubis
A fatty prominence underlying the pubic hair.

## muscular dystrophy
A genetic disease characterized by a wasting away of the muscles.

## mutagens
Agents that cause somatic and germinal mutations.

## mutation
A permanent gene change that is passed on to other generations of cells or organisms.

## myometrium
The muscular wall of the uterus.

## myotonia
Muscle tension.

## natural resources
Resources provided by the environment; nonrenewable resources such as fossil fuels are in finite supply; renewable resources such as water and solar energy are in constant supply.

## natural selection
A process by which the environment favors the survival and reproduction of some members of a species as opposed to others.

## necrophilia
The desire to have sexual contact with dead people.

## nondisjunction
The failure of chromosomes to separate, especially during meiosis.

## nucleic acid
A molecule made up of nucleotides joined together; for example, DNA and RNA.

## nucleotide
A subunit of a nucleic acid containing a molecule of phosphate, sugar, and a base.

## nucleus
A large organelle containing the chromosomes and acting as a control center for the cell.

## oocyte
A germ cell undergoing meiosis in females; for example, primary and secondary oocyte.

## oogenesis
Production of eggs in females by the process of meiosis and maturation.

## organelle
A body within a cell that has a specific structure and function.

## orgasm
Climactic sexual responses including both physical and emotional responses.

## oval opening
An opening between the right and left portions of the embryonic and fetal heart.

## ovarian cycle
The follicular and hormonal changes that occur as the ovary responds to gonadotropic hormones during an approximately 28-day cycle.

## ovarian follicle
Ovarian structure that contains a germ cell in which, the first stage of meiosis occurs in females.

## ovary
Female gonad; that portion of the pistil (female part of flower) that produces the ovules.

## oviducts
Tubes that connect the ovaries and the uterus; these tubes receive the egg following ovulation and are where fertilization occurs.

## ovulation
The release of a secondary oocyte from a Graffian follicle.

## ovules
Particulate-like structures produced by flowers in the ovary that contain the female gamete (egg nucleus).

## oxytocin
A hormone produced by the posterior pituitary that is necessary for milk letdown.

## parturition
Labor, followed by childbirth.

## pedophilia
The desire of an adult to have sexual contact with a child.

**pelvis**
A bony cavity formed by the pelvic girdle along with the sacrum and coccyx.

**penis**
The copulatory organ of males.

**perineum**
The space between the anus and the scrotum in the male and the anus and the mons pubis in the female.

**phenotype**
The appearance of an individual, which is a direct result of inherited genes.

**phenylketonuria**
A genetic disease characterized by the inability to metabolize phenylalanine, leading to mental retardation.

**pituitary gland**
An endocrine gland located at the base of the brain; it is called the master gland because it controls other endocrine glands.

**placenta**
The region where the embryo or fetus receives nutrients and discharges waste.

**plasmid**
Extrachromosomal DNA that occurs in the form of a small ring in bacteria.

**polar body**
Nonfunctioning cell that has little cytoplasm and is formed during oogenesis.

**pollen**
Particulate-like structures produced by flowers that carry the male gamete (sperm nucleus).

**polygenic**
A trait that is controlled by more than two genes.

**postnatal**
After birth has taken place.

**prenatal**
Before birth has taken place.

**primary sex characteristics**
The sex organs of an individual.

**progesterone**
One type of female sex hormone, the other being estrogen.

**prolactin**
A hormone that stimulates the breast to produce milk; also called lactotropic hormone.

**proliferation phase**
That portion of the menstrual cycle when the uterine lining is proliferating under the influence of estrogen.

**prostaglandin**
Chemicals first found in seminal fluid that have many biological effects, including contraction of uterine muscle, so that it can be used to induce abortions.

**prostate gland**
A gland that surrounds the urethra just below the bladder; secretes fluids that are a part of seminal fluid.

**prostitute**
A person who is paid for having sexual contact with another person.

**protein**
A molecule that is made up of amino acids joined together in a specific sequence. All enzymes are proteins.

**protein synthesis**
The process by which protein is made in cells.

**puberty**
That time of life when the sex organs mature and the secondary sex characteristics appear.

**pubis**
The pubic bone, that portion of the hipbone forming the front of the pelvis.

**Punnett Square**
A contrived square that allows the determination of expected ratios of offspring by having all possible sperm fertilize all possible eggs.

**pure dominant**
A genotype having two dominant genes for a characteristic, such as EE.

**pure recessive**
A genotype having two recessive genes for a characteristic, such as ee.

**radiation**
Electromagnetic waves, some of which can increase the incidence of cancer.

**rape**
Force sexual relations. Gang rape: when a number of assailants have sexual contact with one victim. Statutory rape: having sexual contact with a minor.

## recombinant DNA
DNA that carries a new and different portion; particularly *E. coli* plasmid DNA carrying non-*E. coli* DNA.

## refractory period
A period of time after ejaculation when the penis will not respond to sexual stimuli.

## releasing factors
Hormones produced by the hypothalamus that control the production of pituitary hormones.

## reticular activating system
A portion of the reticular formation that extends from the medulla to the thalamus and is believed to alert higher centers.

## Rh factor
An antigen on red cells that can cause a woman to produce antibodies against her baby's blood.

## RNA
Ribonucleic acid; found in molecules that take the genetic message to the ribosomes and transfer amino acids to the ribosomes, designated as mRNA and tRNA, respectively.

## sadist
A person who is sexually aroused by inflicting pain upon a sexual partner.

## scrotum
A pouch of loose skin that contains the testes.

## secondary sex characteristics
All those features that help distinguish males from females other than the sex organs themselves. For example, breasts, beard, musculature, voice, etc.

## secretory phase
That portion of the menstrual cycle when the uterine lining becomes secretory under the influence of progesterone.

## semen
Sperm and seminal fluid combined.

## semiconservative
The DNA duplication process that results in an old strand paired with a new strand; thus, a double helix is formed.

## seminal fluid
The fluid portion of semen.

## seminal vesicles
Small glands that lie at the base of the bladder and secrete fluids that are a part of seminal fluid.

## seminiferous tubules
Long, thin tubules in the testes that produce sperm.

## septicemia
The presence of infectious organisms in the blood.

## sewage treatment plants
Plants that treat fecal matter so it does not contaminate the environment. Primary plants remove solids; secondary plants change solids to chemicals; and tertiary plants prevent these nutrient chemicals from entering nearby bodies of water.

## sex chromosomes
The chromosomes that determine sex (XX in females, XY in males).

## sex-limited gene
A gene whose expression is influenced by the sex hormones of the individual.

## sex-linked inheritance
A somatic characteristic that is inherited by the X chromosome.

## sex-linked recessive gene
A recessive gene that is carried on the X chromosome and controls a somatic characteristic.

## sexual intercourse
Also called copulation or coitus; the act of placing the penis in the vagina.

## sexual reproduction
Reproduction that involves the union of gametes produced by two parents.

## sexuality
Encompasses sex identity, gender role, and sexual conduct.

## sibling
Offspring of the same parents; brothers or sisters.

## sickle cell anemia
A genetic disease characterized by sickle-shaped red cells.

## smegma
A thick, cheesy secretion found under the foreskin.

## sociobiology
The field of biology that applies evolutionary theory to the social sciences.

## sodomy
Usually refers to copulation between males by the anus, but sometimes refers to copulation with an animal.

## somatic
Pertaining to the body, excluding the sex organs.

## somatic mutation
A mutation that occurs in body cells as opposed to germ cells.

## spermatogenesis
Production of sperm in males by the process of meiosis and maturation.

## spermicidal
Capable of killing sperm.

## sterilization
Any process that renders a person incapable of reproducing.

## strand
A term used to designate a nucleotide chain.

## superfemale
A female with more than two X chromosomes; although there is a tendency toward mental retardation, most have no apparent physical abnormalities.

## survival of fittest
The likelihood of better adapted organisms surviving and reproducing.

## Tay-Sachs disease
A genetic disease causing impairment of the nervous system.

## temporal lobes
Lobes on either side of the cerebrum that are believed to inhibit sexual behavior.

## testes
The gonads of the male that develop in the abdominal cavity but descend into the scrotal sacs (scrotum).

## testosterone
The most potent of the androgens, the male sex hormones.

## thalamus
The portion of the brain that passes on sensory stimuli to the cerebrum and therefore is known as the gatekeeper of the cerebrum.

## transcription
The formation of mRNA complementary to a DNA strand; when the code is transcribed into codons.

## translation
The joining of amino acids in the order dictated by the DNA code and mRNA codons.

## transsexual
A person who believes he/she is actually the opposite sex and is trapped in the body of the wrong sex.

## transvestite
A person who likes to wear the clothing of the opposite sex.

## *Treponema pallidum*
The bacterium that causes syphilis.

## *Trichomonas*
Protozoan (microorganism) that causes an infection of the vagina.

## tubal ligation
Cutting of the oviducts, a method of sterilization in females.

## tumescence
The state of being swollen, such as in the case of an erect penis.

## Turner's syndrome
A disease of a female with a single X sex chromosome; these females do not undergo puberty and generally are of subnormal intelligence.

## umbilical cord
A tubular structure that runs between the fetus and the placenta, containing the umbilical vein and umbilical artery.

## underdeveloped countries
Nonindustrialized countries that have a low Gross National Product (GNP) per capita.

## urethra
A tubular organ that conveys urine away from the bladder; also transports sperm in males.

## uterus
Muscular organ, also called the womb, that lies between the bladder and rectum. Embryonic and fetal development occurs in the uterus.

## vagina
Canal leading from the uterus to the vestibule that serves as the copulatory organ in females.

Glossary

**vaginismus**

Involuntary spastic contraction of the muscles about the vagina.

**vas deferens**

See ductus deferens.

**vasectomy**

Cutting of the ductus (vas) deferentia, a method of sterilization in males.

**vasocongestion**

Expansion of an organ or tissue due to the entrance of blood.

**venereal disease (VD)**

A disease acquired by sexual activities.

**voyeurism**

The achievement of sexual gratification by looking at other people in the nude or watching others engage in sexual activities.

**vulva**

The region containing the external genitalia of females.

**XYY male**

A male with the sex chromosomes XYY; characteristics include above average height, persistent acne, and subnormal intelligence.

**zygote**

A cell resulting from fertilization that will develop into the new individual with the diploid number of chromosomes.

# Index

## A

ABO blood groups, 40–41
Abortion, 186–87
  in IUD users, 179
Acne, 96
Acrosome, *12*, 104, 151
ACTH, 89, 116
  in fetus, 166
Adaptation to environment, 212
Adenine, 56, 58, 59
ADH, 87, 89
Adrenal glands, 89, 94–95
Adrenocorticotropin. *See* ACTH
Afterbirth, 169
Agammaglobulinemia, 51–52
*Agapornis* parrots
  behavior of, 216–*17*
Albinism, 66
Allantois, 163
Altruism, 221
Amino acids, 61
Amniocentesis, 15, *16*, *17*, 33,
    37, 43, 156
Amnion, 156, *159*, *163*
Amniotic cavity, *163*
Amniotic fluid, 15, 17, *156*, *159*
Anaphase, *8*
Androgen-insensitivity syndrome,
    230
Androgens, 90–91, 94–95, 104,
    122
  and behavior, 232
  during development, 85–86,
    230–233
  in females, 90, 94–95, 122,
    232
  in sexual disorders, 230–33
Anemia, sickle-cell, 37, 67
Animal behavior. *See* Behavior
Animal contacts, 133
Antibodies, 41, 51, 191, *193*
  in birth control, 186
  following vasectomy, 175
Anticodon, 63
Antidiuretic hormone. *See* ADH
Antigens, 41
  H-Y, 85

ARAS. *See* Reticular activating
    system
Areola, 96, *97*, 153
Artificial insemination, 170–89
Asexual reproduction, *211*
Autosomes. *See* Chromosomes,
    autosomal

## B

Baboon, behavior of, 218, *219*,
    *220*
Baby
  birth of, 166–70
  development of, 156–66
Bacteria, *192*
Baldness, *52*
Bartholin's glands, 145
Bases
  complementary, 54 *(See also
    specific names)*
Behavior, 216–22, 224–34
  and genes, 216
  and hormones, 230–34
  human reproductive, 221–22
  instinctive, 225
  learned, 129, 224–25, 234
  response to stimuli, *224*, 225,
    226
Bestiality, 133
Biochemical genetics, 56–57
Biotic potential, 238
Birth, 166–70
  defects, 159–60
Birth control, 174–87 *(See also
    name of method)*
  after intercourse, 185–86
  effectiveness, *175*
Bisexuality, 131
Bladder, *108*, 119
Blood cells, *37*, 40
  sickle-shape, *37*
  white, *193*
Blood clotting
  in pill users, 178

Blood types, 40–42
  ABO, 40
  combined, 42
  Rh, 41
Brain, 226–30, *227*, *228*, *229*
  and behavior, 224, 226–30
  and erection, 142–43, *144*
  and hormones, 88–*89*
  and lactation, 97–*98*
  male-female, *233*
  and orgasm, 147
Breast, 96–97
  buboes, 201
Bulbocavernosus muscle, 142,
    145

## C

Cancer, 70–75
  in birth control pill users, 178
  lung, *73*
*Candida albicans*, 64
Capacitation, 109, 151
  *in vitro*, 170
Carcinogen, 71
Carrier, gene, 30
Carrying capacity, of
    environment, 238
Cell, *3*
  daughter, 7
  mother, 7
  sex. *See* Gametes
  somatic, 7
Cell division, 6–13. *See also*
    Meiosis and Mitosis
  spindle, 7
  stages, 7, *8*, *10*
Cell fusion, 79
Central nervous system. *See*
    Brain
Centrioles, *8*
Centromere, 7
Cerebrum, *229*
Cervical mucus, 118, 177, 184
Cervix, *113*, 119, 151
  and diaphragm, *180*
  dilation of, 167, 187

Chancres
  hard, 197, *198*
  soft, 201
Chancroid, 201
Childbirth. *See also* Birth
  prepared, 170
Chloasma, 178
Chorea, Huntington's, 35
Chorion, 157, 159, 162, *163*
Chromatid, 7
Chromosomal abnormalities, 14–21
  autosomal, 14–17
  sex, 17–21
Chromosomal inheritance, 13–23
Chromosomes, 3–22, 24
  autosomal, 6
  daughter, 7
  duplicated, 7, 59
  sex, 6, 17, 46
Circulation
  in fetus, *161*
Circumcision
  of penis, *110*
Climacteric, 106
Clitoris, 124, 145, *146*
Cloning, 171
Code, genetic, 61
  faulty, 66
Codons, 62
Coitus. *See* Intercourse
Coitus interruptus, 181–82
Color blindness, 47–49
Colostrum, 97
Complementary bases, 57
Condom, *181*
Contraception. *See* Birth control
Contraceptives
  relative effectiveness of, 175
Copulation. *See* Intercourse
Corpora cavernosa, 142, *143*
Corpus albicans, *115*
Corpus luteum, *115*, 116, 121, 153, 164, 186
Corpus spongiosum, 142, *143*
Cortisol, 89
Cowper's glands, 109, 111, *144*, 145
Crabs, 204, *205*
Cri du Chat, 17, *18*
Cunnilingus, 137
Cytoplasm, 3
Cytoplasmic organelles, *3*, 62
Cytosine, 56, 58, 59

**D**

D & C. *See* Dilatation and Curettage
Deoxyribonucleic acid. *See* DNA
Deoxyribose, 56
DES, 185
Developed countries, 239
Development, 156–66
  embryonic, 162–164
  fetal, 164–66
  of sex organs, 85–86
Diaphragm, *180*–81
Digestion
  in adult, 157
Dilatation and Curettage, 187
Dilation stage of parturition, 167
Diploid
  advantages of, 213
  number of chromosomes, 7
Disease, genetic. *See* Genetic diseases
DNA
  code, 61
  duplication, 59
  recombinant, 76–79, *77*
  structure, 56–*58*
  ladder, *57*
Dominance, gene, 24, 28–29, 33–35
Dominance hierarchies, 220
Double helix, 57
Doubling time
  of population, 238
Douche, 184–85
Down's syndrome, *14*
Drugs
  and birth defects, 159–60
  and pregnancy, 159–60
  and sexual arousal, 230
Ductus deferens, *101*, 107, 175
Duplication, chromosomal, 59, *60*

**E**

E. coli, 77
Ectopic pregnancy, 119
Effacement, *167*
Egg, 6, *12*, 115, 119, 151. *See also* Oogenesis
Ejaculation, 111, 143–45
  premature, 150
Ejaculatory ducts, 107, *144*
Elephantiasis, *203*
Embryo, 121, *156, 163,* 170
  and sex development, 230–34
Endocrine glands, 87–91, *88*
Endometrium, 121
Endoplasmic reticulum, 62

Environment
  and evolution, 212
  and population growth, 243–47
Environmental resistance, 238
Enzyme, 61, 66
Epididymides, 106
Episiotomy, 169
Erectile tissue, 111, 142, *144*, 145
Erection, 110, 142–44
  of clitoris, 145
  of penis, 142
  as reflex, 144
  following vasectomy, 175
Erogenous zones, 137, 225
Erythroblastosis, 42
Estrogen, 118
  effect on behavior, 230, 232–34
  in male, 90, 94–95, 105, 230
  in menstrual cycle, 121
  in the pill, 177
  in pregnancy, 152
  synthetic, 185
Evolution, 211–13
  behavioral, 216–22
  of sexual reproduction, 211–15
Excitement phase, of sexual response, 148
Excretion
  in female, *113*, 124
  in fetus, 157
  in male, 107
Exhibitionist, 133
Exponential growth
  of population, 236
External genitals. *See* Genitals, external
Extraembryonic membranes, *156*–58, 162

**F**

Fallopian tube. *See* Oviduct
Family
  human, 221
Feedback control, 91–92
  in female, 117
  in male, 105
Fellatio, 137
Female reproductive anatomy, 113–25
Female sex hormones, 118
Fertile period, 183–84
Fertility. *See also* Infertility
  of male, 109

Fertilization, *13*, 24, 104, 119, 151–53
  *in vitro*, 170
  water versus land, 215
Fertilized egg. *See* Zygote
Fetal
  circulation, 161
    changes at birth, 169
  development, 164–66
  membranes, 156–58, 162
  sex, 166. *See also* Embryo
Fetishism, 133
Fetus. *See also* Fetal
  digestion in, 157
  excretion in, 157
  respiration in, 157
Flower, parts, *214*
Foam, contraceptive, 182
Follicle, ovarian, *115*, 177
Follicle stimulating hormone. *See* FSH
Follicular phase
  of ovarian cycle, 116
Forebrain, *229*
Foreplay, 136
Foreskin
  of penis, 109
Frogs
  life cycle, *216*
Fruit fly
  population growth, *239*
FSH, 89, 90, 93, 105, 116–17
  and the pill, 177
  in females, 116
  in infertility, 188
  in males, 105
  in menstrual cycle, 116
  releasing factor, 88, 92, *93*, 116
Fungus, 192

G

Gametes, 6, 26, 101. *See also* Egg; Sperm; Gametogenesis
  evolution of, 213–14
Gametogenesis, 6, 9–13, *11*
  in female, *115*–16
  in male, 102–*3*
Gender
  identity, 127, 130
  role, 128, 130
Genes, 2, 24
  and behavior, 216
  dominant, 24
  man-made, 75
  recessive, 24
  sex-linked, 46

Genetic
  crosses, 28
  diseases, 30–43, 46–52 (*See also names of specific diseases*)
    age at onset, 35
    cures for, 77
    dominant, 33–36
    incompletely dominant, 36–38
    polygenic, 42
    recessive, 30–33
    sex-linked, 46–52
  engineering, 79, 171–72
  experiments
    *in vitro*, 75–79
  inheritance
    autosomal, 24–42
    sex-linked, 46–52
  material, 56
  research, 76–90
  traits
    abnormal. *See* Genetic disease
    normal, 28
    variations, 211–13
Genetics, biochemical, 56–90
Genital Herpes, 200, *201*
Genitals. *See* Sex organs
  external
    female, *124*
      infections, *201, 204, 205*
    male, *101*
Genotype, 24–25
  determination of, 24–27
German measles, 160
Germ cells
  in female, 114, *115*
  in male, *103*
Gerontophilia, 133
Glans penis, 109–*10*, *144*, 150
GNP, developed versus nondeveloped countries, 242
Gonadotropic hormones, 87, 90, 92–95
Gonads, 89, 92–93. *See also* Ovaries, Testes
Gonorrhea, 192, 194, 195–97, *195*
  and infertility, 188, 196
  gonococcus
  proctitis, 197
Graafian follicle, *115*
Gross national product. *See* GNP
Guanine, 56, 58, 59
Gulls
  behavior, 217
Gummas, 199, *200*

H

Hair
  axillary, 96
  curly, inherited, *36*
  pubic, 96
Haploid
  number of chromosomes, 9
HCGTH, 153, 163, 170, 186
Hemoglobin
  in sickle-cell anemia, 37, *67*
Hemophilia, 49
Hernia
  inguinal, *107*
Herpes
  genital, 200
  simplex, 200
Heterosexuality, 130, 131
Heterozygous. *See* Hybrid
Hindbrain, *228*
HMG, 188
Homosexuality, 130, 131
  and hormone levels, 232
Homozygous. *See* Pure
Hormonal regulation
  in female, 116–18
  in male, 105–6
Hormones, 85–92, 230–34 (*See also specific names*)
  and behavior, 230–34
  major, 87
  sex, 85
Human
  chorionic gonadotropic hormone. *See* HCGTH
  population growth, 236–38
  reproduction, 85–207
Huntington's chorea, 35
Hutchinson's teeth, 200
H-Y antigen, 85, 233
Hybrid, 24
Hymen, 125, *146*
Hypothalamus, 88, *89*, 91, 105, 116
  and behavior, *229*
  in fetus, 166
  and lactation, *98*
  and pituitary, *89*

I

ICSH, 105
Immunity, 191. *See also* Antigens and antibodies
  as a means of birth control, 186
Implantation, 119, 121, 151, *152*
  ectopic, 119
  following *in vitro* fertilization, 170

Impotency, 150
Incest, 132
Incomplete dominance, genetic, 37
Infectious diseases
    venereal, 191–206
Infertility, 188–89
Inguinal canal, 107
Inheritance, 3–82
    chromosomal, 3–23
    genetic, 24–55
    multifactor. *See* polygenic
    polygenic, 38–43
    sex-limited, 52
    sex-linked, 46–52
Insulin, 76, 77
Intercourse, 136, 137–*38*, 146
    chance of pregnancy, 174
Interphase, *8*
Interstitial cells, 102, 104
Ischiocavernosus muscle, 142, *143*
IUD, 179–80
    side effects, 180

**K**

Karyotype, *4*
Kidneys, 107, *108*
Klinefelter's syndrome, 20, *21*

**L**

Labia majora, *124*
Labia minora, *124*
    sexual response, 145, *146*
Labor, stages of, 166–69
Lactation, 88, 97
Lactotropic hormone. *See* Prolactin
Laparascopy, 170, 176
Law, and sex, 134–35
Lesbianism, 130, 131
    and hormone levels, 232
Lesch-Nyhan syndrome, *50*
Levitor ani muscles, *143*
LGV. *See* Venereum
LH, 89, 90, 93, 104, 105, 116–17
    in females, 116
    in infertility, 188
    in males, 105
    in menstrual cycle, 116
    and the pill, 177
    releasing factor, 88, 92, *93*, 116

Life cycle
    human, *6*
    plants, 214
    sexual, *214*, 215
Limbic system, *229*–30
Lobes of brain, *229*
Luteal phase
    of ovarian cycle, 116
Luteinizing hormone. *See* LH
Lymphatic system, 202
Lymph nodes, 201
Lymphogranuloma venereum, 201

**M**

Male reproductive anatomy, 101–11
Male sex hormones, 91, 104–5
Mammals
    reproductive behavior, 217–22
Mammary glands. *See* Breast
Man-made
    genes, 75
    radiation, 74
Man-mouse cells, 79–80
Marriage, 130–31
Masochism, 137
Masters and Johnson, 148–49
Masturbation, 137
Medulla oblongata, *228*
Meiosis, 6, 9–13
    in female, 115
    in life cycles, 213–14
    in male, 103
    overview, *9*
    stages, *10*
Melanin, 66
Membranes
    extraembryonic, *156*
Menarche, 122
Menopause, 122
Menses, 121, 153. *See also* Menstruation
    in pill users, 177
Menstrual cycle, 120–22
    and ovarian cycle, 121
    regulation, 187
Menstruation
    beginning of, 121
    and birth control pill, 177
    cessation of, in pregnancy, 153
    duration of, 122
    hormonal influences on, 121
Messenger RNA, 62
Metabolic
    diseases, 66
    pathways, 61

Metaphase, *8*
Microsurgery, 189
Milk production, 97, *98*
Miscarriage, 186
    and DES, 185
Mitosis, 6, 7–8, 161
    overview, 1
    stages, *8*
Mongolism. *See* Down's syndrome
Mons pubis, 124
Multifactor inheritance, 38–43
Mutagens, 70
    and infertility, 188
Mutation, 33
    germinal, 70
        in evolution, 211, 213
    somatic, 70
Mytonia, 145, 148

**N**

Natural childbirth. *See* Childbirth, prepared
Natural resources, 244
Natural selection, 212–13
Necrophilia, 133
Nondisjunction, 15, *16*, 19
Nucleic acid
    DNA, 56–58
    RNA, 58–59
Nucleotides
    in DNA, *56*
    in RNA, *58*
Nucleus, *3*
Nursing. *See* Lactation

**O**

Obscene phone calls, 133
Oocyte, 115, 151
Oogenesis, *11*, 115
Oral contraceptive, 177–79, 185–86
Orgasm, 142–48
    dysfunction, 150
Orgasmic phase, 148
Oval opening, *161*
Ovarian cycle, 116, 121
    and menstrual cycle, 121
Ovaries, 114
Oviducts, 119, 151, 176
Ovulation, *115*, 117, 119, 122, 151
    day of, 123, 183–84
    induced, 170
    multiple, 170

and the pill, 177
and rhythm method of birth
    control, 183–84
Ovum. *See* Egg
Oxytocin, 88, 97–98, 167

**P**

Parturition, 166–70
Pedigree chart, 30, *31*
    for color blindness, *49*
Pedophilia, 133
Peeping Tom, 133
Pelvic girdle, 98, 99, 169
Pelvis, *98*, 99
Penis, 109–11, 142–44
    erection of, *110*, 142
    and use of condom, 181
Perineum
    female, 145
    male, 142
Pesticides, 72
Phenotype, 24–25
Phenylketonuria. *See* PKU
Pheromones, 225
Pill, birth control, 177–78
    side effects, 178–79
Pituitary gland, 88–*90*, 91
    activity in lactation, *98*
    hormones of, *90*
    relation to hypothalamus, *89*
PKU, 32–33, 66
Placenta, 121, 153, *159*
Plasmid
    experiments, 76–79
Plateau phase, 148
Pleasure center, 230–*31*
Pollution, 246
Polygenic inheritance, 38–43
Population
    age profiles, *243*
    growth rates, 240
    human, 236–248
    increase, 237
Pornography, 133
Pregnancy, 151–53, 174
    ectopic, 119
    hormonal activity in, 97, 152
    prevention of, 185. *See also*
        Birth control
    rate, 174
    signs of, 153
    tests, 153
    tubal, 119
Prenatal
    development, 161–66
    diagnosis, 42–43
Primary sex characteristics

Progesterone, 94–95, 116–18,
    122
    as birth control medication,
        186
    in birth control pills, 177
    in menstrual cycle, 121
    in pregnancy, 152
Prolactin, 87, 97
    and infertility, 188
Proliferation phase
    of menstrual cycle, 121
Prophase, *8*
Prostaglandins
    during birth, 166
    to induce abortion, 185, 187
    in seminal fluid, 109, 151
Prostate gland, 109
Prostitutes, 132
Protein
    structure of, 61
    synthesis of, 61–*65*
Puberty, 92–93
Pubic hair, *96*
Punnett Square, *13*, 26
Pure
    dominant, 24
    recessive, 24

**R**

Radiation
    and infertility, 188
    man-made, 73–75, 160
    natural, 72–75
Rape, 132
Recombinant DNA. *See* DNA,
    recombinant
Refractory period
    in female, 148, 149
    in male, 111, 145, 148
Releasing factors, 88, *93*, 105,
    116
Reproduction, 85–207
    asexual, 211
    in the laboratory, 170–71
    sexual, *6*
        evolution of, 213–15
Resolution phase, 148
Respiration, 157
Reticular activating system, *228*
Rh factor, *41*–42
Rho Gam, 41
Rhythm method of birth control,
    183–84
Ribonucleic acid. *See* RNA
Ribose, 59
Ribosomal RNA. *See* Ribosomes
Ribosomes, *3*, 62
Ring doves, behavior of, *234*

RNA, 59
    messenger, 62
    ribosomal, 62
    transfer, 62

**S**

Sadism, 137
Safe period
    for intercourse, 183–84
Salpingitis, 196
Salting out, 187
Scrotal sacs, 102
Scrotum, 102
    and varicose veins, 188
Secondary sex characteristics.
        *See* Sex characteristics
Secretory phase
    of menstrual cycle, 121
Semen, 109, 111, 145
    and coitus interruptus, 181–82
Seminal fluid, 108, 151
Seminal tubules, 102–*3*
Seminal vesicles, *101*, 108
Septicemia, 197
Sertoli cells, 103, 186
Sewage treatment plants,
    247–*48*
Sex
    characteristics
        primary, 85, 101, 113
        secondary, 85, 92–99
            after sterilization, 174
    chromosomes, 6, *13*, 17–21,
        86
        abnormalities, 17–21
    drive, 128, 232
    hormones, 85–99
        cellular activity, 86
        female, 91, 117–18, 122,
            123
            in birth control pill, 177
        male, 91, 105–6
    organs. *See also* Ovaries and
            Testes
        in female, 113
        in fetus, 85–87, 166
        in male, 101–2
    role. *See* Gender role
Sex-limited traits, 52
Sex-linked inheritance, 46–52
Sexual
    activities, 136–38
    behavior, biology of, 224–35
    conduct, 127, 128–29,
        131–39
    diseases, 191–206
    dysfunction, 150–51

intercourse, 137–*38*, 146
offenses, illegal, 134–35
partner, 131–33
reproduction
  biological advantages, 213
  evolution of, 211–22
response, 148–49
Sickle-cell anemia, *37*, 67
Skin color, 38–40
Smegma, 110
Smoking
  and birth defects, 159
  and cancer, *73*
  and the pill, 178
Sociobiology, 215
Sodomy, 132, 134, 137
Sperm, 6, 12, 104, 151. *See
    also* Spermatogenesis
count, 109
Spermatic cords, 107, 175
Spermatids, 103
Spermatocytes, 103
Spermatogenesis, *11*, 102–4
Spermatozoa. *See* Sperm
Spermicidal cream, foam, jelly,
  182
Spindle apparatus, 7, *8*
Spirochete, syphilis, 197, *198*
Sterility, 102
Sterilization, 175–77
  hysteroscopic, 176
Stickleback fish
  reproductive behavior, *226*
Superfemale, 19
Syndrome (*See specific names*)
Syphilis, 197–200
  congenital, 200


**T**

Tay-Sachs, 33
Technology, 245
Telophase, *8*
Template, 60, 62
Tes-Tape, 184
Testes, 102–5
Testosterone, 91, 94–95, 105
  as means of birth control, 186
Thalamus, *229*
Thalidomide, 159
Thromboembolism, 178

Thymine, 56, 59
Transcription, gene, 62, *63*
Transfer RNA, 62
Translation, gene, 62–*64*
Transsexuals, 130
Transvestites, 131
*Treponema pallidum, 198*
Trichomonas, 203
Triplet code
  of DNA, 61
Tubal ligation, 176–*77*
Turner's syndrome, 19, *20*


**U**

Umbilical cord, 153, 160, *161*,
  169
Underdeveloped countries, 239
Uracil, 58, 59
Urethra, 107–8, 142, *143*
Urethritis, in male
  gonococcal, *195*
  nongonococcal, 202
Urogenital system, 158
  in females, 124
  in males, 107, *108*
Uterine aspiration, 187
Uterus, 113, 119, *120*, 146,
    151, 167
  in abortion, 187
  contractions of, in labor, 166
  and IUD, 180
  in menstrual cycle, 121–22
  at orgasm, *146*–47
  during pregnancy, 121,
    *165–66*


**V**

Vagina, *113*, 123
  acidity of, 123
  as birth canal, 169
  infections of, 203
  as organ of copulation, 146
  at orgasm, 146–47
Vaginismus, 151
Vaginitis, 203
Varicocoele, 189
Vas deferens. *See* Ductus
  deferens

Vasectomy, 175–*76*
Vasocongestion
  at orgasm, 142, 147
Vasopressin, 87, 88. *See also*
  ADH
Venereal diseases, 191–206
Venereum
  granuloma, 203
  lymphogranuloma, 201, *202*
Vernix caseosa, 166
Vestibular bulbs, 145
Vestibule, 124
Viruses, *192*
Voice, 96
Voyeurism, 133
Vulva, *124*


**W**

Warts, genital, 204, *205*
Water cycle, *244*
Womb. *See also* Uterus
  artificial, 171
World growth rate, 237


**X**

X chromosome. *See* Sex
    chromosomes
  and sex-linked genes, 46–52
X-ray. *See* Radiation


**Y**

Y chromosome. *See* Sex
    chromosomes
Yeast infection of vagina, 203
Yolk sac, 163


**Z**

Zero population growth. *See*
    ZPG
Zona pellucida, 104, 151
ZPG, 242
Zygote, 6, 24, 119, *152*, 157,
    162
  in life cycles, 213–15